Subjected to Science

The Henry E. Sigerist Series in the History of Medicine
Sponsored by The American Association for the History of
Medicine and The Johns Hopkins University Press

*The Development of American Physiology: Scientific Medicine in
the Nineteenth Century* by W. Bruce Fye

*Save the Babies: American Public Health Reform and the
Prevention of Infant Mortality, 1850–1929*
by Richard A. Meckel

Politics and Public Health in Revolutionary Russia, 1890–1918
by John F. Hutchinson

*Rocky Mountain Spotted Fever: History of a Twentieth-Century
Disease* by Victoria A. Harden

*Quinine's Predecessor: Francesco Torti and the Early History of
Cinchona* by Saul Jarcho

The Citizen-Patient in Revolutionary and Imperial Paris
by Dora B. Weiner

*Subjected to Science: Human Experimentation in America before
the Second World War* by Susan E. Lederer

Subjected to Science

Human Experimentation in America
before the Second World War

Susan E. Lederer

The Johns Hopkins University Press

Baltimore and London

This book has been brought to publication with the
generous assistance of the American Association for the
History of Medicine.

The Johns Hopkins University Press
2715 North Charles Street
Baltimore, Maryland 21218-4319
The Johns Hopkins Press Ltd., London

ISBN 0-8018-4820-2

Library of Congress Cataloging-in-Publication Data will be
found at the end of this book.
A catalog record for this book is available from the British
Library.

For Mark

Contents

Illustrations

Acknowledgments

Many librarians and archivists provided assistance with this project. I am indebted to Karen Hall, whose inventiveness made the days spent at the College of Physicians and Surgeons at Columbia University a pleasure. At the Rockefeller Archives, Carolyn Kopp and Lee Hiltzik speeded my research, as did the staffs of the Alan Mason Chesney Archives at the Johns Hopkins Medical Institutions, the Harvard Medical School, the Library of the University of California at San Francisco, and the College of Physicians of Philadelphia. Joan Echtenkamp Klein and Mark Mones provided extraordinary assistance with the Walter Reed materials at the University of Virginia. Finally, I owe special thanks to Dana Zazo and Esther Dell at the George T. Harrell Library of The Pennsylvania State University College of Medicine for their aid, which went above and beyond the call.

The idea for this book began in Ronald Numbers's living room. He may not recall the moment, but I remember it well, along with his unwavering guidance and support.

A number of people have contributed substantially to this book. Judith Leavitt, Guenter Risse, Todd Savitt, John Parascandola, Pat Ward, Ellen More, and Charlotte Borst challenged my thinking about human and animal experimentation. My colleagues at Hershey—David Barnard, Al Vastyan, K. Danner Clouser, David Hufford, and Eric Juengst—greatly encouraged my work, and June Watson provided unfailing and invaluable assistance. I am especially grateful to Jon Harkness and to Jackie Wehmueller of the Johns Hopkins University Press for their critical readings. Naomi Rogers, who read the entire manuscript with her characteristic insight, energy, and forthrightness, has been a constant friend.

Portions of essays previously published in the *Bulletin of the History of Medicine* and *Isis* are incorporated in this work, and I am grateful to the Johns Hopkins University Press and the University of Chicago Press for permission to use them.

My family has learned a great deal about the history of human experimentation during the writing of this book. Gregory and Eric could spell antivivisection from an early age. Jeff, Margot, and David Lederer helped locate sources, and my mother-in-law, Margaret Lederer, translated Spanish documents relating to the vivisection of criminals into English for my use. Mark has helped in more ways than I can count, and I dedicate this book to him.

Introduction

Human guinea pigs. For many Americans, these words suggest disturbing images of men, women, and children exploited in the name of medical science. The disclosures in recent years of federally sponsored research involving American citizens—the Tuskegee Syphilis Study, a forty-year study of untreated syphilis in African-American men; the nerve and mustard gas tests conducted during World War II on American soldiers; and in 1993, reports of radiation experiments on dying patients, pregnant women, and mentally retarded children during the Cold War—have intensified many of the negative associations with human experimentation.

At the same time, these disclosures have raised questions about the development of ethical standards for human experimentation. What, if any, were the rules for research involving human beings in the 1940s and 1950s? What ethical standards should we use to evaluate these earlier experiments? Perhaps most important for policy makers, is it fair to apply the ethical standards of the 1980s and 1990s to researchers working in the 1930s and 1940s, when, presumably, different ethical norms were in place?

Part of the problem in answering these questions has been a reluctance to look seriously at the conduct of human experimentation before World War II. With few exceptions, historians and bioethicists have assumed that research involving human subjects, especially nontherapeutic experiments, occurred only rarely before the war and that the moral problems posed by human experimentation concerned few physicians or the lay public.[1] The modern history of human experimentation, according to these scholars, begins with the Nuremberg Code, developed in 1946 as part of the prosecution of Nazi physicians for war crimes and crimes against humanity.[2] Because the Nuremberg Code and its emphasis on the voluntary consent of the individual subject represents a milestone in the history of human experimentation, understanding the development of ethical standards in the years before World War II is not only important but essential.

This book examines the public and professional debates over human experimentation in the first four decades of the twentieth century. During this period, the moral issues raised by experimenting on human beings were most intently pursued by the men and women committed to the protection of laboratory animals, the American antivivisectionists. Already devoted to saving dogs, cats, and other animals from the vivisector's knife, antivivisectionists warned that the replacement of the family physician by the "scientist at the bedside" would inspire nontherapeutic experimentation on vulnerable human beings. That animal protectionists would embark on a defense of the human subjects of medical research may surprise many readers, because today animal and human experimentation are distinctly different enterprises. In the late nineteenth century, however, the two activities were seen as intimately related. In fact, it was an antivivisectionist sympathizer, British playwright George Bernard Shaw, who first introduced the term "human guinea pig" in the early twentieth century, to make clear the vivisector's equation of human and animal subjects.[3]

Spurred by newspaper reports of physicians who injected hospital patients and orphans with the germs of infectious diseases, American antivivisectionists and their allies accused the medical profession of placing scientific goals before patient welfare. The controversy over "human vivisection," conducted in the pages of popular magazines and in the committee rooms of the United States Senate, prompted leaders of the American medical profession to consider regulating human experimentation thirty years before the Nuremberg Trials. Why prominent medical researchers and the leaders of the American Medical Association decided not to do so at that point is explored in detail in this book.

Some readers may find the references to vivisection puzzling. *Vivisection* literally means cutting into a live organism, animal or human. A surgical operation on a human patient, as surgeon William Williams Keen pointed out in 1914, is literally a human vivisection. In the late nineteenth century, however, the word *vivisection* was used to denote any experimental manipulation. Despite critics like Keen, who protested that only a small percentage of animal vivisections (6% in Britain, where statistics had been available since 1876) involved cutting a living organism, most Americans used *vivisection* and *experimentation* interchangeably.[4] *Human vivisection*, on the other hand, was used to describe only those experiments on human beings undertaken not to benefit an individual subject but to provide medical information. As physician and vivisection-reformer Albert T. Leffingwell explained, human vivisection could be distinguished from those acceptable experiments undertaken to benefit patients. "In the practice of medicine," Leffingwell observed, "there must always be a 'first time' when a new method of medical treatment is employed, a new operation performed, a new remedy employed. Whether the procedure pertain to medicine or surgery, so long as the amelioration of the patient is the one purpose kept in view, *it is legitimate treatment.*"[5]

Use of the term *human vivisection* to refer to nontherapeutic experiments on human beings continued well into the 1930s. In the 1932 film based on H. G. Wells's novel *The Island of Dr. Moreau*, American audiences heard the actor Richard Arlen express outrage at the "human vivisections" conducted in the House of Pain. In 1933, playwright Sidney Howard, who adapted both *Arrowsmith* and later *Gone with the Wind* for the screen, used the term *human vivisection* in *Yellow Jack*, a Broadway play and subsequent film based on Walter Reed's yellow fever experiments in Cuba.[6] This book continues this usage; the terms *human vivisection* and *nontherapeutic experimentation* are used interchangeably.

Human vivisection must be understood in the larger context of animal protection. The American antivivisection movement has not attracted the serious historical attention it deserves. A history of the antivivisection movement in the twentieth century, for example, remains to be written. In addition to exploring the connections between human and animal protection, this book considers some of the questions raised by the controversy over human vivisection. Did American physicians routinely perform nontherapeutic experiments on their patients? Who served as the subjects of these experiments and what risks did they encounter? Did physicians obtain permission for experimentation from patients or their families? What were the limits on human experimentation in this period and how were they enforced?

My research reveals both the range and the complexity of experimental encounters between American investigators and their subjects, as well as the politics of medical research that governed professional responses to the accusations of "murder in the name of science." In his history of the Tuskegee Syphilis Study, historian James H. Jones maintains that in the 1930s, there was "no system of normative ethics of human experimentation that compelled medical researchers to temper their scientific curiosity with respect for the patient's rights."[7] Contrary to Jones's claims about a "formless relativism" in human subjects research, my work demonstrates that even before 1930, researchers observed limits in their experiments with human subjects. Although lacking enforcement policies and far from perfect, ethical guidelines influenced the conduct of research with both human and animal subjects in the decades before World War II. At no time were American investigators free to do whatever they pleased with their human subjects. Neither their peers nor the public would have stood for reckless experimentation that endangered human lives. Thus, many researchers expressed their apprehension about risking patient welfare in tests of new drugs and procedures, mindful of the difficulties—professional and legal—that could arise if a patient were seriously injured. Jones's claims must be reconsidered in light of such findings.

In the first four decades of the twentieth century, the moral problems posed by infecting human beings with yellow fever or withholding orange juice from asylum infants until they developed scorbutic lesions were discussed not only in medical journals but also in the popular media— newspapers, fiction, and films. In his Pulitzer Prize-winning novel *Arrowsmith* (1925), Sinclair Lewis, for example, described a confrontation between some potential human subjects and a medical researcher from the thinly disguised Rockefeller Institute for Medical Research. Sent by his superiors to test a newly developed serum on a plague-infested island in the West Indies, Martin Arrowsmith explains that a control group will be necessary to determine if the serum is effective against the disease. His plan to administer the experimental injection to only half the population, while sternly depriving the rest, provokes hostility and disbelief. "There isn't much I can do now—these doctor Johnnies have taken everything out of my hands," the island's governor bitterly exclaims, "but as far as possible I shall certainly prevent you Yankee vivisectionists from coming in and using us as a lot of sanguinary . . . corpses."[8] Arrowsmith is able to perform the experiment only after Oliver Marchand, a black physician, makes "his people" on the nearby island of Carib available for the test.

Fiction, of course, teaches its own truths. The novel does offer some voices seldom heard in the history of American medical research. Lewis allows the potential research subjects—at least the white and wealthy ones—to express their disgust for the experimenter's proposal and to refuse to participate. The voices of the Carib natives, "volunteered" by their physician, are not heard; how they viewed their participation in the study is not addressed by the author. These are voices and stories that deserve our consideration. Unlike the experimenters whose names and exploits are chronicled in the medical literature, the men, women, and children who served as research subjects have been largely mute, anonymous, or simply invisible. Although we cannot easily restore the stories of these silent subjects to the history of medical research, we can get closer to their voices and experiences by paying close attention to the situations in which human experimentation occurred and to the social arrangements between experimenters and their subjects. These are some of the stories I have sought to tell.

Subjected to Science

Chapter One

"The Sacred Cord": Doctors, Patients, and Medical Research

In the late nineteenth century the embrace of experimental medical science transformed the American medical profession. Knowledge acquired in the laboratory and the clinic established a new basis for therapeutic practice and paved the way for reforms in medical education. Allegiance to scientific medicine and laboratory research became a source of professional legitimacy for American physicians, who redefined the ideal physician from a practitioner, whose authority stemmed from the exercise of clinically informed judgment, into a scientist, the possessor of specialized knowledge gained from experiments on animals and human beings.[1]

What principles would guide physicians in their investigations, and who would be the subjects of their experiments? In 1907 the eminent clinician William Osler maintained that "the limits of justifiable experimentation upon our fellow creatures are well and clearly defined. The final test of every new procedure, medical or surgical, must be made on man," he informed the Congress of American Physicians and Surgeons, "but never before it has been tried on animals."[2] Once animal experiments established the "absolute safety" of a new drug or procedure, he explained, physicians who obtained "full consent" were justified in applying the new therapy to their patients. "We have no right to use patients entrusted to our care for the purpose of experimentation unless direct benefit to the individual is likely to follow. Once this limit is transgressed," he solemnly observed, "the sacred cord which binds physician and patient snaps instantly." Using healthy volunteers in medical experiments created different responsibilities for physicians than investigations involving patients. In his 1907 address, Osler contended that as long as participants had "full knowledge of the circumstances" and willingly submitted to the experiment, studies on volunteers were not only permissible but praiseworthy. Although enthusiasm for science produced a few "regrettable transgressions," he argued that these rare cases did not detract from the incalculable benefits of experimentation to medicine.[3]

Osler's observations on the requirements for ethical human experimentation, which echoed the opinions of many other physicians in the late nineteenth and early twentieth centuries, bear scrutiny. How did the duties of the physician in the experimenter-subject relationship differ from those in the traditional doctor-patient relationship? Did clinical investigators routinely meet the conditions of therapeutic benefit and full consent of patients when they conducted experiments? How did physicians define *therapeutic benefit* and *consent*? Did volunteers possess "full knowledge of the circumstances" when they agreed to participate in medical research? How did the medical profession respond to "regrettable transgressions" involving human subjects?

This chapter examines the changes in medical science that increased the number of experiments involving both patients and volunteers after 1870 and explores the ways in which American physicians reconciled the demands of scientific medicine with the traditional responsibilities of the doctor-patient relationship, as well as the unease that the prospect of a scientist at the bedside created for American patients. Medical responses to experiments, both celebrated and infamous, involving human subjects constituted an implicit standard for handling the issues of therapeutic benefit for the participant, injury to the subject, the willingness of the investigator to "go first," and the consent of the patient or volunteer.

Developments in the medical sciences created new opportunities and demands for human experimentation. The new disciplines of pharmacology, bacteriology, and immunology stimulated considerable experimentation on human beings beginning in the late nineteenth century. The discovery of new technologies, including the x-ray and the stomach tube, fostered a growing number of experiments involving both sick individuals and those identified as normal by investigators. The reorganization of the hospital and, perhaps equally important, the epistemological shift that made knowledge acquired on hospital patients applicable to private patients, together encouraged physicians to undertake investigations involving patients. One indication of the growth of medical research was the appearance in the 1890s of three new journals devoted to original medical research. Although William Henry Welch, who started the *Journal of Experimental Medicine* in

1896, expressed concern that the enterprise would founder from lack of contributors, he was soon overwhelmed by papers. The *Journal of Medical Research*, founded that same year, gave American investigators another forum for reporting original research involving both animal and human subjects, as did the *American Journal of Physiology*, which began publication in 1898.[4]

The science of bacteriology engendered substantial experimentation on human beings and animals. Although initially indifferent, if not hostile, to the germ theory of disease, American physicians responded with enthusiasm to Robert Koch's announcement of the discovery of the tubercle bacillus in 1882.[5] Hunting the bacillus, "bacteriomania," became the order of the day. In addition to the idea that a specific microorganism caused a particular disease, Louis Pasteur and especially Robert Koch provided physicians with the techniques for bacteriological research. Isolating and identifying a disease germ under the microscope was the first step. After growing the microorganism in a pure culture, the physician needed to use the germ to produce the disease in a healthy organism.

The use of human beings to confirm that a microbe caused a particular disease or to demonstrate the mode of transmission was a harsh legacy of the germ theory of disease. Unable to find a suitable animal model in which to study the disease, physicians turned to human subjects. Before the discovery that monkeys could be infected with syphilis and gonorrhea, the search for the microbes of venereal disease prompted more than forty reports of experiments in which individuals were inoculated with the suspected germs of gonorrhea and syphilis.[6] In 1895 New York pediatrician Henry Heiman, for example, described the successful gonorrheal infections of a 4-year-old boy ("an idiot with chronic epilepsy"), a 16-year-old boy (an "idiot"), and a 26-year-old man in the final stages of tuberculosis.[7] In addition to using infants, dying patients, and mentally impaired individuals to demonstrate the pathogenic effect of microorganisms, physicians used their own bodies for bacteriological experiments. Many of these experiments, ironically, involved investigators who categorically rejected the idea that a microscopic organism alone could cause complex human diseases. One of the most famous self-experiments was conducted by the German chemist Max von Pettenkofer, who decided to challenge Koch's claim that cholera vibrio alone could cause the disease. In 1892 Pettenkofer swallowed a pure culture of cholera bacilli, suffered only a mild case of diarrhea, and continued to maintain his claim that the germ alone did not produce cholera.[8]

For other physicians, the identification of a microbe as the causative agent of a disease was the first step toward developing both diagnostic tests and vaccines to treat and prevent disease. Much of the vaccine testing was performed on children, because they lacked previous exposure to infectious diseases. Although vaccination for smallpox had been introduced in the late eighteenth century, physicians continued to study the nature and mechanism of immunity to the disease. In 1895 Walter Reed and George M. Sternberg, for example, investigated the immunity produced by smallpox vaccination in children at several Brooklyn orphanages.[9] Evaluating the quality of a new vaccine often entailed risks for the children who participated in testing it. In order to establish that a vaccine protected a child against smallpox, some physicians injected children with active smallpox virus after vaccinating them against the disease.[10]

Physicians also attempted to develop vaccines for such childhood diseases as measles, chickenpox, scarlet fever, and tuberculosis. Often such experimentation proceeded with the permission of parents. Seeking a means to prevent the spread of scarlet fever, one Chicago physician in 1900 attempted to immunize the two brothers of a child already suffering from the disease. "With the consent of the father," W. K. Jaques inoculated the boys with scales of the disease.[11] The possibility that an experimental vaccine might pose a greater threat than the natural acquisition of a disease obviously troubled physicians. Parental permission for an experimental vaccine helped to alleviate medical concerns about bad outcomes. In 1912, when Colorado physician Gerald Webb developed a vaccine for tuberculosis, the prospect of "inoculating the non-infected" with the germs that cause tuberculosis distressed him. Only after "a distinguished scientist dying of tuberculosis" offered the Colorado physician an "unusual opportunity" did Webb attempt the vaccination of the scientist's two children, aged 9 months and 3 years.[12]

Bacteriology and immunology fostered many experiments involving human beings. The development of pharmacology similarly spurred drug testing on humans and animals. Before 1860, as historian John Harley Warner has shown, therapeutic practices were grounded in the principle of specificity. Physicians prescribed medical therapy that matched the specific characteristics of the individual patient and the social and physical environment of the patient. In the decades after the Civil War, medical commitment to therapeutic specificity weakened, supplanted by a belief that therapeutic knowledge obtained on one group of patients could appropriately be applied to other human beings.[13]

In the late nineteenth century the isolation of new chemical com-
pounds and improvements in the purification of drugs offered physicians a
variety of new drugs that required testing on both animals and human
beings. Reports in 1884 of the anesthetic properties of cocaine apparently
fostered widespread self-experimentation among "willing medical students
and intelligent surgeons." One surgeon to attempt cocaine anesthesia was
William Halsted. With his colleague Richard Hall, Halsted used cocaine on
himself and on medical students at Roosevelt Hospital in New York City. As
a result of their studies, Hall, Halsted, and some of their assistants became
addicted to the drug. Halsted's drug addiction nearly derailed his career in
academic medicine. During his hospitalization for cocaine addiction, the
young surgeon received morphine (then often prescribed as a treatment for
both alcohol and drug addiction). Although he subsequently enjoyed a
brilliant career as professor of surgery at the Johns Hopkins Hospital, Halsted apparently struggled with opiate addiction for the rest of his life.[14]

In some cases, pharmacologists moved to human beings once extensive
testing on animals had demonstrated the safety and efficacy of a new compound. For example, seeking to develop a purgative that could be administered intravenously, pharmacologist John J. Abel and his colleague Leonard
Rowntree systematically studied a wide variety of phthalein derivatives on
dogs. After isolating a chloride preparation with no toxic properties, they
studied the action of the compound on a series of human patients.[15] The
discovery of vitamins and the understanding of nutritional deficiency diseases that came in the first two decades of the twentieth century entailed
testing on both normal and ailing human subjects. At the same time, the
revival of interest in chemotherapy similarly fostered trials on both animals
and humans.

New technologies, including the gastric tube, the x-ray, and the electro-
cardiograph, gave physicians the opportunity to obtain information about
human physiology, normal and abnormal, without causing serious discomfort and risks. Introduced as a therapeutic measure for gastrointestinal disease, the stomach tube enabled physicians to study gastric secretion and
digestion in sick and healthy human beings. Before 1880, for example, the
study of digestion in children was confined to experiments on animals and
dead infants. The stomach tube could be used, even in very young infants,
to answer questions about infant feeding. After 1896 the development of
the x-ray enabled unprecedented visual information about the interior of
the human body. Most applications of the rays were therapeutic or diagnostic in nature, but some physicians used x-rays to study physiological pro-

cesses in healthy adults and children. In addition to x-raying the fetus in utero, physicians studied the sequence of bone development in infants and children.[16] In order to determine the normal size and shape of the infant stomach, for example, Godfrey Pisek and Leon Theodore LeWald administered bismuth to babies aged 2 days to 20 months. They performed serial x-rays to study the behavior of the stomach with different foods, the passage of food, and the motility of the stomach at various times.[17]

Changes in the social organization of American medical care facilitated the experimental study of human health and disease. In the decades after the Civil War, the American hospital was transformed from a largely custodial institution for the indigent into a scientific institution attracting patients from the middle and upper classes. Beginning in the 1880s Americans witnessed a tremendous increase in the number of hospitals and hospital beds. In 1873 the first American hospital survey reported only 178 hospitals (including institutions for the mentally ill) and fewer than 50,000 beds. By 1909 the number of hospitals (excluding hospitals for the mentally ill) had expanded to 4,359 institutions with 421,065 beds.[18]

The hospital offered physicians more than the opportunity to heal the sick. A small number of elite physicians advocated the "scientific use of hospitals," both to increase medical knowledge and to create better-trained physicians.[19] By establishing specially equipped hospitals or hospital wards, physicians could study aspects of specific diseases or clinical problems. When the sixty-bed Rockefeller Institute Hospital opened in 1910, it was the only such institution devoted entirely to clinical research. In conjunction with the Rockefeller Institute for Medical Research, clinical investigators could extend their observations and tests to patients specially selected to complement the research mission of the institution.[20] Few hospitals could match the funding, special equipment, laboratories, and staff of the Rockefeller Hospital; but advocates of hospital research noted that with improved recordkeeping and standardization of hospital routines, even general hospitals could be advantageously harnessed for research purposes: "The general scientific atmosphere created by a body of men and women seeking to solve medical or surgical problems will usually result in the highest type of clinical work, to the benefit of the patient."[21]

Using the hospital scientifically did little to ease traditional anxieties about experimenting doctors. For most of the nineteenth century, suspicion that indigent patients would become the unwitting subjects of therapeutic experimentation in life and the objects of dissection after death persisted among many Americans. Although physicians conceded that patients were potentially at risk from experimenting doctors, they insisted that the mistreatment of hospital patients in both teaching and research was considerably more common on the other side of the Atlantic. American physicians who had studied in the Paris clinical schools in the first part of the nineteenth century were convinced that human life was little valued in French hospitals. Parisian patients were "mostly looked upon as good subjects for the dissecting knife," observed one American physician.[22] In the second half of the nineteenth century, American physicians who pursued postgraduate medical study in the hospitals and clinics of Vienna, Berlin, and other European cities continued to criticize the treatment of patients in Continental hospitals.[23] These physicians and surgeons recalled their distaste for the attitudes displayed by German physicians toward their patients. "They would attempt things that in most other countries would be considered unjustifiable," the surgeon J. M. T. Finney observed. "Though the results were fairly satisfactory, the human element was largely lacking. The patient was something to work on, interesting experimental material, but little more."[24]

In the last quarter of the nineteenth century, the importation of the German medical model into American medical education, the calls for the "scientific use of hospitals," and several well-publicized cases of hospital experimentation intensified concern about the treatment of patients in American hospitals. The folklorist Gladys-Marie Fry traced the origins of an African-American oral tradition about "night doctors" to the years between 1880 and World War I, when large numbers of blacks migrated to northern cities. Fears that "night doctors" would kidnap black people for experimentation and dissection flourished in the African-American community.[25] Distrust of hospitals would continue to grow among both the rich and poor, argued one correspondent to *Outlook* magazine in 1900, until the public was assured that "the hospital is for man, not vice-versa, for the benefit of patients, not data."[26] Research-oriented physicians contended that the hospital could serve both functions. Reconciling the needs of patients and the demands of research, however, was not easily accomplished. The absence of injury to a patient or research subject, the potential for therapeutic benefit, the physician's willingness to participate in the study, and the consent of the patient or volunteer were criteria in professional and lay determination of what was ethical human experimentation.

An experiment on a "feeble-minded" woman at the Good Samaritan Hospital in Cincinnati illustrates some of the problematic features of hospital experimentation in the last quarter of the nineteenth century. In 1874

Mary Rafferty, a 30-year-old Irish woman employed as a domestic servant, entered the hospital. Physicians diagnosed the infected ulcer on her scalp as cancerous and attempted to treat her condition surgically. Realizing that little could be done to save her life, physician Roberts Bartholow initiated a series of experiments that involved the insertion of needle electrodes into her exposed brain substance. His graphic research report detailed her discomfort from the studies:

> When the needle entered the brain substance, she complained of acute pain in the neck. In order to develop more decided reactions, the strength of the current was increased by drawing out the wooden cylinder one inch. When communication was made with the needles, her countenance exhibited great distress, and she began to cry. Very soon, the left hand was extended as if in the act of taking hold of some object in front of her; the arm presently was agitated with clonic spasm; her eyes became fixed, with pupils widely dilated; lips were blue, and she frothed at the mouth; her breathing became stertorous; she lost consciousness and was violently convulsed on the left side. The convulsion lasted five minutes, and was succeeded by a coma. She returned to consciousness in twenty minutes from the beginning of the attack, and complained of some weakness and vertigo.[27]

As Rafferty's condition worsened, her physicians abandoned further experiments. After she died, a few days later, Bartholow concluded from the autopsy that, although electrodes had damaged portions of her brain, her death had resulted from cancer.

Bartholow's published report of his experiments in cerebral localization prompted British investigators, including the neurologist David Ferrier, to criticize such reckless use of living human beings.[28] American physicians expressed similar reservations about Bartholow's conduct and the abuse of the doctor-patient relationship that ended with Mary Rafferty's death. A resolution at the 1874 American Medical Association meeting condemned Bartholow's experiments, calling them "so in conflict with the spirit of our profession, and opposed to our feelings of humanity that we cannot allow them to pass unnoticed."[29]

The chief issue taken with the experiment on Mary Rafferty was the injury that she sustained as a result of the insertion of the electrodes. Injuring patients in the name of science was unacceptable to American physicians. It violated one of the cardinal duties of the physician—to avoid doing harm. While defending his actions, Bartholow conceded that further studies with the needle electrodes would be "in the highest degree criminal" but only in light of the knowledge he had gained from the electrode studies of Rafferty's brain: "I can only now express my regret that facts which would further, in some slight degree, the progress of knowledge were obtained at the expense of some injury to the patient."[30]

The Rafferty case also raised the question of consent by the subject. Bartholow insisted that the Irish woman had not been the subject of involuntary experimentation. Although "feeble-minded," Mary Rafferty had given "cheerful assent" to his proposals. Some critics challenged the value of permission given by a patient with her limited mental ability. "Had Mary been other than 'feeble-minded,'" another hospital patient, "not of the Good Samaritan Hospital," wrote to the *Philadelphia Medical Times*, "perhaps she might have been in doubt as to whether the hospital in which these things were allowed was not a misnomer."[31] Even though he failed to address the issue of consent from a feeble-minded person, Bartholow's frank apology and assurance that further experimentation would not be undertaken helped to placate some—but not all—of his critics.[32]

In the late nineteenth century patient consent was a complicated and often ambiguous feature of experimentation, both therapeutic and nontherapeutic. Just as hospital patients served as "clinical material" in the teaching of medical students, they were expected to agree to being part of a trial of a new drug or procedure when their physicians believed that it promised some benefit to them or at least did not harm them. "Like the men who have lived in times of political crisis and turmoil," Boston physician Charles Francis Withington explained in his 1886 Boylston Prize–winning essay on the relations between hospitals and medical education, "their environment was their misfortune."[33] If a physician's research involved such benign procedures as the collection of anthropometrical tracings or the taking of blood pressure readings, performing studies on hospital patients without consent was not morally problematic. "If the physician were to ask these things as a favor, few, if any, patients would refuse him"; Withington observed, "and if as a matter of convenience he takes them as a right, no harm was done."[34] When physicians undertook research involving discomfort and risk to the patient without the promise of therapeutic benefit, they were obligated to inform patients and obtain their consent.

American responses to the clinical trials of two English physicians and to the cancer-grafting experiments of French and German doctors illustrate the complex intersection of patient consent and therapeutic benefit. In 1883 William Murrell, a lecturer in *materia medica* at Westminster Hospital, administered nitrite of sodium to eighteen outpatients. Although he followed the recommended dosages, Murrell used a highly purified form of the drug, which produced severe and distressing reactions in the patients. Murrell's associate, Sydney Ringer, a physician at University College Hospital of London, then tested the drug on cats and frogs and verified the highly toxic nature of the purified drugs at the standard dosages. After repeating their tests of sodium nitrite and other drugs on several additional sets of hospital patients, they published an account of their clinical trials that aroused considerable comment in England. Public criticism of the Ringer-Murrell studies prompted an inquiry by the Censor's Board of the Royal College of Physicians, which subsequently exonerated both physicians of professional misconduct.[35]

In the United States, physician responses to the Ringer-Murrell controversy were mixed. Charles Withington pronounced their use of hospital patients to determine the physiological response to drugs "an egregious usurpation" of the patient's "right to immunity from experiments" that had no therapeutic application. Such tests were permissible only when investigators obtained patient consent prior to the trials: "If the experimenters wished to investigate the physiological action of the drug they should have called for volunteers; they had no right to make any man the unwilling victim of such an experiment."[36] Although he accepted the distinction between therapeutic and nontherapeutic experimentation, an American defender of the English physicians disputed any characterization of the drug testing as nontherapeutic. Murrell's decision to administer the drug to selected outpatients, argued physician John V. Shoemaker, was inspired by a promising report in the medical literature of the drug's efficacy in the treatment of epilepsy. Administering the drug only to those patients who fit the diagnostic criteria insured that these patients could anticipate a therapeutic benefit from the drug. (The Censor Board cited this argument in their decision to exonerate Murrell's conduct.)[37] Lamenting that opponents' attacks on Murrell's experiments as "wanton" had not been confined to the laity, Shoemaker contended that Murrell deserved the "thanks of the profession for his [therapeutic] demonstrations, rather than virulent abuse; for with a cessation of 'experiment' the progress of medicine must also cease."[38]

Issues of therapeutic benefit and patient consent were also features of American medical responses to reports of cancer-grafting experiments by French and German physicians. In 1891, in an effort to determine whether cancer was contagious, French physician Victor Cornil analyzed breast tissue samples from two women who received cancer grafts during surgical removal of their breast cancer. In a paper, Cornil described how a "foreign surgeon" amputated a woman's breast containing an enormous tumor. While the patient remained under chloroform, and without her consent, he sectioned a piece of the tumor and implanted it into her healthy breast. After two months, the implant, which had grown to the size of an almond, was extirpated by the surgeon for microscopic examination. The same surgeon duplicated this procedure on another patient. This second graft also produced a nodule. The patient refused further surgery and disappeared from the surgeon's purview.[39]

When Cornil's report was presented to the Académie de Médecine, the assembled physicians and surgeons denounced the experiments as criminal and refused to discuss the scientific aspects of the two cases.[40] In his defense, Cornil explained that he had not performed the cancer grafts; he had only analyzed the data. Failing to use the information, Cornil insisted, would have been unethical. American physicians rejected his explanation as "pure sophistry." Placing abstract knowledge above patient welfare compromised the medical profession, observed one medical writer: "And questions which require for their solution the infliction of needless suffering on human beings, must wait until a proper opportunity for their solution presents itself."[41] One such opportunity was the route taken by Chicago surgeon Nicholas Senn. In 1901, in an effort to resolve the question of cancer's contagiousness, he inoculated himself with cancerous tissue obtained from one of his patients. (He did not develop a tumor.)[42]

American physicians soon learned that Cornil was not the first to attempt cancer grafting in human beings. An official inquiry in July 1891, undertaken by the Prussian minister of religious, educational, and medical affairs, established that German surgeons Eugen Hahn and Ernst von Bergmann had performed similar surgical cancer grafts, but with intentions that were in part palliative.[43] In order to satisfy a hopelessly ill patient who demanded an operation, the surgeons performed an operation that included implanting cancerous tissue in a woman's breast, "an experiment harmless to her and bearing on questions of eminent practical and scientific importance not otherwise capable of solution."[44] The physicians did not expect their patient to live very long and so felt that implanting the cancer during the surgery could not harm her and could answer the vitally important questions of whether cancer could be transported in the body.

This argument had been clearly articulated by the French physiologist Claude Bernard. "The principle of medical and surgical morality," he explained in *An Introduction to the Study of Experimental Medicine* (1865), "consisted of never performing on man an experiment which might be harmful to him to any extent, even though the result might be wholly advantageous to science, i.e. to the health of others."[45] At the same time, experiments on people condemned to death (either by civil authorities or by disease) were "wholly permissible." Like the French helminthologist C. Davaine, who fed larva-infected sausage to a woman soon to be executed in order to see whether worms would develop in her intestines after her death, the German surgeons had not compromised the welfare of their subject by the cancer implant.[46] The absence of injury to patients may have been more important to the German physicians than the fact that patients consented. Even in cases in which patients permitted dangerous, nontherapeutic experiments, one medical writer observed, physicians were obligated to place individual well-being above scientific gain: "We feel called upon to caution scientific investigators that in dealing with human beings they are treading upon dangerous ground, even when acting with the patient's consent."[47]

Unlike Cornil's experiments, the German grafts received support from American physicians. Hahn's patients reportedly experienced less pain and did not complain of the surgery, and the grafts "were performed with the full consent and understanding of the patients, whose condition was not rendered in any sense more unfavorable by the operation."[48] Permission of the patient, absence of injury, and therapeutic benefit (the placebo operation) combined to exonerate the conduct of the German physicians.

What physicians understood by the words "full consent and understanding" is less clear than the circumstances in which they solicited patient permission. The surgeon William B. Coley, who developed a new treatment for malignant tumors, explained that he obtained the consent of patients before administering his experimental injections to produce "an artificial erysipelas." Coley described how one patient, a 46-year-old German cigarmaker suffering from a large sarcoma of the back and groin, initially resisted the injection. "After some deliberation he consented, and on the 21st of April, 1892 I began inoculations."[49] The responses to Robert Koch's announcement of a cure for tuberculosis illustrates the ways in which patients, families, and physicians negotiated the decision to try new therapies. In their published case reports, the American physicians who administered tuberculin, Robert Koch's reported cure for tuberculosis, emphasized the patient's role in the decision to receive the treatment and the uncertainty of the outcome. (Tuberculin did not turn out to be a cure, but was later used successfully to diagnose tubercular infection.) "At the urgent request of relatives, treatment was decided upon with the clear understanding of the fact that the case did not belong to the class of incipient cases in which complete recovery could be looked for with a certainty."[50] When President Benjamin Harrison obtained a small vial of Koch's lymph for Charity Hospital in New Orleans, physician Joseph Jones did not employ the lymph because, he explained, "without exception the patients under my treatment and care in the wards of the Charity Hospital declined to submit to this mode of treatment."[51] The experimental nature of the therapy and the uncertainty of the outcome fostered respect for the patient's right to refuse the lymph. No American legislature, however, went as far as the Prussian government, which, in 1891, enacted a regulation that insured that tuberculin would "in no case be used against the patient's will."[52]

Patients retained in principle the right to decline innovative or risky medical therapies. Some physicians, concerned that extremely ill patients were vulnerable to novel medical recommendations, warned their colleagues against the "temptation" of championing a procedure that could "have no other advantage than to enhance the operator's reputation for boldness."[53] In 1888, gynecologist James W. Etheridge advised his colleagues that the consent of the patient—"obtained without direct or indirect coercion"—was essential for "the most difficult, dangerous and formidable procedure in operative obstetrics," performing a caesarean section. The reference to coercing a patient's decision to undergo a risky procedure suggests that physicians did in fact pressure patients to accede but that such coerced consents did not protect a physician when a bad outcome occurred. When a procedure became both less risky and more routine, physicians did not solicit patient consent. In the case of caesarean section, for example, Etheridge predicted that the time would come when such consultations between women and their doctors would no longer be necessary: "The woman shall not be permitted to elect as freely as she must be allowed to do so at present."[54]

What did physicians tell patients or their families in order to enlist their support? We have little access to the communications between doctor and patient. For most nineteenth-century physicians, disclosure and truth-telling were secondary to the professional responsibility for patient welfare. The decision to inform a patient about the seriousness of his or her medical condition exemplifies professional priorities in the nineteenth century. In his influential 1803 work on medical ethics, the English physician Thomas Percival argued that the patient's right to the truth was "suspended and even annihilated" if it adversely affected the patient, the patient's family, or the community.[55] Percival's vision of medical ethics exerted a profound influence on the American medical profession. When the newly established

American Medical Association adopted a code of ethics in 1847, the membership echoed Percival's views on truth-telling, noting that "the life of a sick person can be shortened not only by the acts, but also by the words or the manner of a physician." The "sacred duty" of the physician was to avoid those disclosures which could discourage or depress a patient. Not all physicians embraced the notion of benevolent deception. Worthington Hooker, the only American physician to publish a monograph on medical ethics during the nineteenth century, criticized the AMA's stance on truth-telling in the doctor-patient relationship. Conceding that lying benefited some patients, Hooker maintained that "the good, which may be done by deception in a *few* cases, is almost as nothing, compared with the evil which it does in many cases."[56] Most American physicians remained unconvinced by Hooker's arguments, and continued to practice deception in the interests of their patients.

The conviction that deception was more beneficial than full disclosure was challenged in 1903, when Boston physician Richard Clarke Cabot reported the results of his comparative study on truth and falsehood in medicine. After having practiced deception and limited disclosure with his patients, Cabot attempted providing patients and their families a "true impression" of the patient's condition. Although his explanations did not necessarily entail the full details of the etiology, pathology, course, and prognosis of the illness, Cabot sought to provide information sufficient for patients and families to understand the nature of the illness. Truth-telling, he found, not only benefited individual patients, who with their families exhibited a capacity to rise to a difficult occasion, but enhanced public confidence in the medical profession.[57]

Few American physicians were persuaded by Cabot's demonstrations of the "astounding innocuousness" of the truth. "Perhaps the safest generalization about medicine" in the late nineteenth century, bioethicists Ruth Faden and Tom Beauchamp have persuasively argued, "is that although routine consent to consequential interventions such as surgery existed, practices of benevolent deception and nondisclosure shaped the professional norm of standard practice, and benevolent deception in the obtaining of consent was not unusual."[58]

In addition to benevolent deception, physicians were motivated by self-interest when enlisting patient consent for therapy and experimentation. Some investigations were not possible without the cooperation of patients or subjects. The patient's "willingness to observe directions to the strictest letter" was essential to the outcome of the experiments.[59] In their published reports, physicians sometimes recorded how patient resistance created obstacles in research. "Induced to make some experiments with [nutritional] injections into the rectum of a negro" in 1901, Philadelphia physician Albert Bernheim described how the "healthy mulatto" followed all his instructions until he attempted to introduce a stomach-tube. Although the subject "would not allow it" at first, the physician eventually overcame his objections.[60] In a study of the spinal fluid in patients with syphilis, physicians performed lumbar punctures to obtain the necessary fluid "if the patient would submit."[61] The experimenter-subject relationship was shaped by negotiations between investigators and their subjects. Subjects exercised some control, albeit limited, over what the experimenter did to them. They were not simple victims of an experimenter's ambition.

We know very little about the circumstances in which physicians overcame objections to a research request. Some patients clearly took part in experiments without their knowledge, or in the belief that the experimental procedure was part of their treatment. In his 1904 study of hookworm infection, one southern physician, Claude Smith, explained that his subject believed that the placement of soil containing hookworm larva on his foreskin was a preparation for the circumcision procedure he had requested. "The patient seemed to have an idea that it was some medicine preparatory to the operation as nothing was said to him about it." After four minutes, the patient remarked "that the prepuce felt as if a fly was crawling over it, and a minute or so later said that it felt as if needles were sticking in it."[62]

Overcoming objections was more difficult with some patient populations. Using children and the inmates of mental institutions often required considerable patience and ingenuity. Some questions could not be answered with these often noncompliant populations. The "mental or physical states" of the female patients at the Connecticut Hospital for the Insane, F. G. Benedict explained, precluded an accurate collection of urine over twenty-four hours.[63] Biochemist Otto Folin encountered similar difficulty with urine collection when he organized a clinical laboratory at the McLean Hospital for the Insane.[64] Collecting such body fluids as blood and saliva from the insane also posed problems. University of California investigator John Albert Marshall noted that after he had explained his project "certain inmates gladly cooperated" with his efforts to study saliva.[65] Eight of his 104 patients remained uncooperative. (He did not explain how he acquired saliva from these reluctant subjects.)

Using institutionalized infants and small children presented different challenges for investigators. Whereas physicians relied on compliance (even if achieved through deception) when they performed such procedures as spinal puncture on adults, juvenile subjects needed only to be restrained long enough to obtain spinal fluid. Because young children would not urinate on command, physicians studying nitrogen excretion in normal children inserted catheters, held in place by strips of adhesive plaster.[66] Most accounts of the problems in studying orphans and hospitalized children did not include gaining permission from parents or guardians. Pediatricians were more likely to thank the medical directors of orphanages, who "graciously furnished the material" for study than to acknowledge that they obtained permission from parents.[67]

In the early twentieth century, a growing number of lawsuits over unauthorized surgical procedures prompted surgeons and hospital administrators to formalize the process of obtaining patient consent. Although oral agreements and implied consent remained legally valid, written consent forms were increasingly viewed as a form of additional protection for surgeons.[68] "It is becoming a common practice of some people, especially the poor and more ignorant classes, to hold surgeons to an unreasonable accountability for their conduct of their cases," observed the authors of a guide to hospital management. Obtaining written permission for surgical operations in hospitals afforded some protection to surgeons when a case ended badly and "some venal lawyer looking for a fee happens to gain the ear of the family of the patient."[69] As more middle-class patients entered the hospital, written consent forms also signaled that hospitalization in itself did not license a physician or surgeon to undertake any measures deemed medically appropriate.

Fears of unauthorized surgery were not new in American medicine. In the mid-nineteenth century, the widespread introduction of anesthesia into American medical practice had invoked the specter of involuntary surgery.[70] But complaints about surgeons who acted against their patients' wishes increasingly filled court dockets. Perhaps the best-known case, the 1914 suit *Schloendorff v. Society of New York Hospital*, involved a New York woman who consented to an exploratory abdominal operation but insisted that no surgical procedure be performed. After her surgeon removed the fibroid tumor discovered during the examination, she brought suit against the hospital where she had undergone surgery. Justice Benjamin Cardozo ruled that the hospital as a charitable institution was not liable for the actions of the staff, even as he affirmed the patient's role in surgical decisionmaking. "Every human being of adult years and sound mind has a right to determine what shall be done with his own body"; Cardozo argued, "and a surgeon who performs an operation without his patient's consent commits an assault."[71] The possibility of legal action encouraged pathologists and hospital administrators to urge physicians to obtain written consent from families of the dead before conducting post-mortem examinations.[72] Although the process took several decades, the courts increasingly upheld the right of a patient's family to give formal consent for operations on the body after death.[73]

Few American patients sought redress in the courts for damages sustained from involuntary experimentation, and few American physicians were subjected to criminal prosecution for the unauthorized use of patients in nontherapeutic research.[74] Nonetheless, fear of legal problems may have constrained American investigators. The prospect of damage suits resulting from experiments involving patients made some American physicians envious of the less restrictive climate of German medicine. "It is fortunate," one American physician observed about tuberculin testing, "that the 'lymph' is being tested among Germans on German patients, for certainly America would never allow this amount of experimentation involving death in some instances, without what might become troublesome investigations."[75]

American law did not forbid experimentation, but judges expected physicians to experiment only when they knew that a good outcome for the patient would ensue. Although in theory a physician was not liable for the failure to effect a cure, departing from standard practice placed the burden for an improved result on the physician. One legal opinion rendered in the late nineteenth century illustrates how physicians could be liable for a bad outcome of an innovative therapy. In the 1871 *Carpenter v. Blake* case, the physician argued that his unorthodox procedure to correct a dislocated shoulder represented innovation rather than negligence. The court, however, ruled that any deviation from standard practice that lacked the approval of respectable practitioners was not acceptable when it did not benefit the patient.[76]

American physicians learned from medical journals of the successful prosecutions of several eminent European physicians. In 1880 Gerhard Armauer Hansen, co-discoverer of the leprosy bacillus, lost his license to practice medicine after he was charged with deliberately infecting the eye of a female hospital patient with a culture of leprosy bacilli.[77] Another case profiled in American medical journals involved the other discoverer of the leprosy bacillus, German bacteriologist Albert Neisser. In the early 1890s, Neisser, who also discovered the gonococcus, tested a newly developed syphilis vaccine on three young girls and five female prostitutes. In 1900,

these syphilis studies prompted attacks against Neisser in the German legislature and culminated in his criminal prosecution. Antisemitism may have
played a role in Neisser's conviction, for which he was fined three hundred
marks.[78] In Italy, a physician who successfully inoculated an elderly man
with malaria in 1903 was prosecuted by the civil authorities in Rome and
received a reprimand for exceeding the boundaries of acceptable research.[79]

Some American physicians noted their concern about the possibility of
a bad outcome from an explicitly experimental procedure. Injuries to subjects could lead to the abrupt end of a research program, emotional strain,
and even potential legal problems. When Isaac Abt's experimental injections of sterilized gelatin into two boys and a "feeble-minded" 4-year-old
girl produced "alarming symptoms of prostration and collapse," he decided
against using children in such studies and to confine future testing to rabbits.[80] In 1912, when A. J. Rongy, an attending gynecologist at Jewish Ma-
ternity Hospital in New York, began his experiments to induce labor in
pregnant women, he was uneasy, "realizing the gravity of such experiments
in a public hospital in this city." Rongy and his staff proceeded cautiously
with the fetal serum. "We were fully aware that any untoward accident
would interrupt all our work and in addition we would have to face serious
consequences."[81] In spite of his uneasiness and the uncertain outcome of
the use of the serum, Rongy asked only one patient whether she had any
objection to the use of the serum. A relative of one of the nursing staff, the
pregnant woman left the decision to the doctor, who gave her the serum.

One way physicians assuaged patients' or volunteers' fears about harm
in research was to experiment on themselves. Although not always possible,
the obligation to try a new drug or procedure on oneself (or one's pet) before
applying it to patients was an accepted feature of medical research in the
mid-nineteenth century. The introduction of anesthetics, for example, fostered considerable self-experimentation with ether and chloroform before
physicians administered the drugs to patients.[82]

Unwillingness to try a new remedy on oneself or one's family before
applying it to patients continued to be cause for criticism in the late nineteenth century. When Robert Koch's 1891 announcement of a new therapy
for tuberculosis prompted considerable clinical testing, one American physician explained that a doctor's reluctance to apply tuberculin to his own
family was unprofessional. "If he were unwilling to administer the lymph to
one of his own family, why should he consider it good practice to inject the
lymph into other invalids just as dear to their families or friends?"[83] By the

same token, the self-experiments that assured the safety of an experimental vaccine for pneumonia insulated physicians from charges of reckless experimentation when they cautiously applied their vaccine to patients.[84]

Experimenting on oneself or one's students and colleagues did offer some advantages. Colleagues and medical students were readily available for experiments and they did not require elaborate explanations of the goals, needs, and risks of the research. Individuals acquainted with laboratory technique could adjust more quickly to the demands of research apparatus. As educated participants, they could also provide more detailed and meaningful observations of their experiences. As Francis G. Benedict, director of the Carnegie Nutrition Laboratory in Boston and a leading researcher in the field of nutrition, explained in 1910: "All of the subjects were engaged in scientific work in the laboratory and were thoroughly familiar with the methods of experimenting and the object of research. Their intelligent cooperation was thus assured."[85]

The most famous self-experiment in the twentieth century was the successful demonstration by U.S. Army physician Walter Reed and the other physicians of the Yellow Fever Board—James Carroll, Jesse Lazear, and Aristides Agramonte—of the transmission of yellow fever by mosquitoes. Although Reed did not actually experiment on himself, his name became a symbol for the heroic self-sacrifice of scientific physicians.

The acquisition of Cuba on the heels of the Spanish-American War intensified American interest in yellow fever. Disease outbreaks threatened the American troops occupying the island as well as the restoration of political, economic, and moral order to the island under American rule.[86] In 1900 Surgeon General George Miller Sternberg organized a medical commission headed by Walter Reed to investigate yellow fever in Cuba. The Yellow Fever Board's research involving human subjects implicated the Aedes aegypti mosquito as the insect vector and facilitated an effective sanitary program to control the disease in Havana and, later, in the Panama Canal Zone.

Because there was no animal model in which to study the disease, efforts to establish the transmission of yellow fever required human subjects. The deliberate infection of healthy human beings with yellow fever involved significant risks. The disease often resulted in death, and physicians could do little for yellow fever patients but offer supportive care. The Yellow Fever Board's proposal to expose healthy human beings to the disease was not lightly undertaken. Both personal concerns and professional considerations influenced the decision of the research team to begin with self-experimentation and later to execute with American soldiers and Spanish volunteers formal contracts that outlined the risks and compensation to the subjects.

Self-exposure to "loaded mosquitoes" was the first step. Agramonte's previous exposure to yellow fever made him ineligible for the experiment, but Carroll, Lazear, and Reed, all nonimmunes, agreed in principle to test the mosquito hypothesis on themselves. According to James Carroll, it was his idea that the investigators begin with their own bodies.[87] Eager to resolve the mosquito question, Carroll and Lazear started to experiment while Reed was away in Washington. After applying an infected mosquito to himself, Carroll developed a severe attack of yellow fever, from which he recovered. Also bitten by an infected mosquito, Lazear died in September 1900.

Why Reed did not participate with Carroll and Lazear remains unclear. Immediately after the members of the board had agreed to the self-experimentation, Reed returned to Washington. Although Reed's biographers have suggested that the Surgeon General ordered Reed back to Washington, no surviving documents support this theory. James Carroll later contradicted the claims that Reed was ordered to return by the military authorities, insisting that Reed was free to return to Washington at will.[88] In any case, after Lazear's death and Carroll's narrow escape, Reed decided against self-experimentation and took steps to avoid contracting the disease. "Perhaps I owe my life to my departure from Cuba," he confided to a friend, "for had I agreed to be bitten along with the others—Being an old man, [he was 49] I might have been quickly carried off."[89]

Lazear's death did not deter several American soldiers who offered to serve as research subjects. Concern about exposing additional human beings to the risks of yellow fever prompted the unusual step of written contracts with the subjects. The contracts outlined the risks of participation in the study as well as the benefits (including good nursing care). Although the American soldiers who took part in the experiments received no immediate financial compensation, the Spanish volunteers received money for participating and a cash bonus if they developed the disease. A grant from the military governor of Cuba, Major General Leonard Wood, provided funds for setting up the experimental research station Camp Lazear and for compensating the volunteers. With the approval of the Spanish consul, Reed restricted participation to those over the age of twenty-four, the Spanish age of consent. Concerns about safety led Reed to insist that no one older than forty be allowed to participate, because of the greater risk to individuals in this age group.

The offer of one hundred dollars in gold, together with free medical care, and an additional hundred dollars if the subject contracted yellow fever, attracted many of the newly arrived Spanish immigrants. So appealing was the offer that some of the immigrants not chosen "almost wept."[90] Those chosen signed the following statement, available in both Spanish and English:

> The undersigned understands perfectly well that in case of the development of yellow fever in him, that he endangers his life to a certain extent but it being entirely impossible for him to avoid the infection during his stay in this island, he prefers to take the chance contracting it intentionally in the belief that he will receive from the Reed Commission the greatest care and the most skillful medical service.[91]

These written contracts perhaps exaggerated the inevitability of natural infection with yellow fever and underplayed the danger to life that yellow fever posed, but they marked a significant departure in the history of human experimentation.

The extraordinary choice to use written contracts may have been influenced by Surgeon General Sternberg. This possibility has received little attention from historians.[92] In May 1900 Sternberg wrote to Aristides Agramonte about the importance of determining whether the infectious agent of yellow fever was present in the blood. Experiments conducted in Vera Cruz in 1885 had failed to resolve the question of whether yellow fever could be transmitted through inoculations of blood from a person sick with the disease. "If you have an opportunity to repeat these experiments and settle this important matter in a definite way," the surgeon general advised Agramonte, "you will bear in mind the fact that they should not be made upon any individual without his full knowledge and consent."[93]

Sternberg had personal experience with human experimentation. In the 1880s, unable to pursue his interest in yellow fever and malaria, he undertook a series of investigations with the newly discovered germ of gonorrhea. Persuaded that Albert Neisser's gonococcus did not cause the disease, Sternberg proposed several inoculation experiments at a San Francisco hospital. He soon learned that "the courage of some of the gentlemen who had consented to the experiment at first had failed them."[94] After the defection of all but one young man, a medical student from Baltimore,

Sternberg was induced to participate when he discovered that his colleague had decided to experiment on himself. "With this example before me I could not do less than join in the experiment," he candidly observed, "although I confess that I did so with some hesitation, notwithstanding the negative results which I had previously obtained in a similar experiment." The three men inserted cylinders of cotton saturated with the fluid gonorrheal culture into their own urethras for several hours. None of the subjects developed gonorrhea.[95]

After this brief foray into the bacteriology of the venereal diseases, Sternberg resumed his research in yellow fever. He closely followed medical developments related to the understanding of the disease. When Italian bacteriologist Giuseppe Sanarelli announced in 1897 that he had discovered the bacillus of yellow fever, Sternberg was one of the first to publish his rejection of Sanarelli's germ. In order to buttress his claim for the role of his bacillus in yellow fever, Sanarelli maintained that he had produced yellow fever in five patients.[96] Sternberg was present at the 1898 meeting where Johns Hopkins clinician William Osler challenged a characterization of Sanarelli's experiments as "simply ridiculous": "To deliberately inject a poison of known high degree of virulency into a human being, unless you obtain that man's sanction, is not ridiculous," Osler argued, "it is criminal."[97] Familiarity with the Sanarelli experiments may have inspired Sternberg to avoid similar pitfalls in his yellow fever research program.

Sternberg's interest in and his advice about insuring the knowledgeable participation of volunteers need not detract from Reed's role in making the decision to adopt written agreements with the yellow fever subjects. Certainly Reed's anxiety about research that risked serious disease and possible death for the volunteers influenced the adoption of written contracts. It may also have helped to assuage any lingering guilt about his own failure to take part in the experiments. At the Pan-American Medical Conference in Havana in February 1901, where he was criticized by a Cuban physician for the human experiments, Reed informed the assembly that he believed that no one appreciated the difficult position in which he found himself or the moral uncertainty that beset his path.[98] Without an animal model for the disease, Reed argued, experimentation on human beings became absolutely necessary. The experiments on the research team and the intelligent consent of the other participants, he claimed, had allayed the anxiety created by deliberately infecting human beings with a dangerous disease.

That Reed hoped to avert the criticism sparked by Sanarelli's human experiments is clear from the attention he directed to his published papers.

In addition to obtaining signed permission forms from the volunteers, Reed made certain that reports of the yellow fever cases in medical journals included the phrase "with his full consent." There was only one exception. In the first published announcement of the documentation of the mosquito transmission of the disease, Reed asked that Sternberg omit the words "with his full consent" to the description of Carroll's and Lazear's cases, because the absence of these words from another case (the case of T. C. Y.) "might attract attention and lead to the inference that his inoculation was done without his consent."[99] After Reed's death in 1902, Sternberg continued to emphasize the voluntary nature of the yellow fever studies. All his published reports stressed that volunteers were "fully informed" of the risks and the benefits of participation in the yellow fever studies.[100]

Given the politically explosive situation in Havana, Reed and his superiors may have hoped to avert local charges of exploitation of the Spanish volunteers. The use of written agreements, the promise of gold, and limiting participation to adults, however, did not prevent several Havana newspapers from attacking the "horrible" use of "unsuspecting" immigrants in the studies.[101] Fortunately for the researchers, for the research subjects, and for the success of the program, all of the volunteers except Lazear recovered from their bouts with Yellow Jack. In a subsequent experiment conducted by the Yellow Fever Board, however, the research-related deaths of a 25-year-old Army nurse, Clara Maass, and two Spanish nonimmune subjects ended efforts to produce an immunizing serum against the disease.[102] The "fatal termination" of the three cases not surprisingly produced a shortage of additional volunteers and a "panicky feeling" toward the experiments, "intensified by the sensational and distorted statements in one of the local Spanish papers."[103]

Despite these attacks, Reed received lasting acclaim for demonstrating the mosquito to be the vector of yellow fever. His "untimely death" from a ruptured appendix in 1902 may have robbed him of being the first American to receive a Nobel Prize in medicine, but his experiments remained models.[104] Like Louis Pasteur, who risked much when he administered his experimental rabies vaccine to a child, Reed made a lasting contribution to medical knowledge. His experiments resolved the question of yellow fever transmission. As historian Gerald Geison has suggested, dangerous human experimentation, therapeutic or nontherapeutic, has been more easily forgiven if the clinical gains were great and the experimenter turned out to be right.[105]

Self-experimentation and the concern that volunteers be "fully informed" helped to exonerate physicians who risked the well-being of their subjects, but when a Brooklyn physician announced that he had infected a young woman with the germ of bovine tuberculosis, the fact that she had given her consent in writing did not protect him from professional and public scorn. In 1902 George D. Barney informed newspaper reporters of startling experiments with bovine tuberculosis. Like Walter Reed, Barney obtained written permission from his human subject for the experiment to demonstrate that bovine and human tuberculosis were the same disease. Unlike the physicians in Cuba, Barney did not perform an initial experiment on himself. Even though a French physician Paul Garnault had publicly inoculated himself with the germ of bovine tuberculosis in an attempt to determine whether tuberculosis in cattle could be transmitted to human beings, Barney rejected this step.[106] Instead, in the presence of the Brooklyn Commissioner of Deeds, Barney instructed Miss Emma King to sign a statement indicating her agreement to be inoculated and absolving Barney of blame if she did indeed develop tuberculosis. King's participation attracted considerable newspaper coverage, including reports that the Brooklyn Board of Health would not interfere because Barney had obtained the prior approval of his subject. At the same time Barney reported that his injections had produced tuberculous symptoms in the young woman, he also announced his "cure" for the disease and cited a 92 percent success rate in curing tuberculosis.[107]

Emma King committed suicide the summer following the experiment.[108] The story of Barney's experiment and its unhappy sequel led some observers to reflect on the ethics of human experimentation. Refuting any parallel between King's "alleged inoculation with consumption" and the case of "the two young doctors in Havana who lost their lives by experimentation with yellow fever germs upon themselves," one newspaper critic insisted that a physician had no right to subject a patient to such risks, even with the consent of the patient.[109] Barney's desire for notoriety and his quackish claim of a cure for tuberculosis earned the scorn of medical writers, who also stressed the poor scientific design of Barney's study and allowed that only self-experimentation might have redeemed the escapade: "If the experimenter had experimented upon himself the case would have had at least a better moral aspect and the opportunities for obtaining anything of value from the results could not have been any worse."[110]

Self-experimentation did not always possess a "better moral aspect." The desire for notoriety undermined medical and lay respect for medical martyrdom. When another Brooklyn physician informed newspapers of his willingness to be vivisected for scientific purposes, the "would-be martyr" was criticized by his colleagues.[111] In 1902 John F. Russell offered his own body to physicians for a period of one year for the purposes of scientific experimentation. When the medical staff of a New Jersey hospital accepted his proposal, Brooklyn's district attorney threatened to prosecute anyone who laid a scalpel on the doctor. The chief of staff at Bushwick Central Hospital informed newspaper reporters that the hospital would not only care for his family and pay all expenses during his year of vivisectional experimentation but would also "guarantee his family a sufficient sum for its future maintenance" in the case of his death.[112]

The activities of Barney and Russell did not diminish the traditional association of experimentation with reckless innovation or quackery that proponents of clinical research hoped to undermine. In the first part of the twentieth century the word *experiment* continued to be avoided. "Be careful never to speak of anything you do for a patient as an experiment or merely to gratify curiosity," advised D. W. Cathell in the 1906 edition of his enormously popular guide to medical practice, "for every body is more or less opposed to physicians' 'trying experiments' upon themselves or theirs."[113]

Trying experiments on patients and healthy volunteers was acceptable to American physicians if it met certain conditions. Prior experimentation on animals and the willingness to use a new drug or procedure on oneself or one's family were important features of acceptable human experimentation. The issue of therapeutic benefit, the absence of injury to the participant, and the consent of the individual, however problematic in practice, also influenced medical evaluations of experiments involving patients and other volunteers. For physicians like Osler, the limits of human experimentation were clearly defined, and the "sacred cord" that bound physicians and patients remained intact.

The advent of scientific medicine and the transformation of the physician into a scientist at the bedside alarmed some critics. Both medical and lay observers voiced concerns about the implications of scientific medicine for medical practice and the doctor-patient relationship. Critical of the overemphasis on bacteriology in the medical curriculum, an Iowa physician expressed his reservations in verse: "Science still stops to reason and explain / Art claps the finger on the bleeding vein."[114] In 1906, former president Grover Cleveland, who claimed to speak for the great majority of patients, noted that although the public welcomed the tremendous advances in medical science, "we do not like to think of our doctors as veiled prophets or mysterious attendants, shut off from all sick-bed comradeship except as such comes through cold professional ministrations, and irrespective to our need of sympathetic assurance."[115]

American antivivisectionists made even more radical claims. As part of a crusade to limit animal experimentation, they focused on the deleterious effects of laboratory science on the practice of medicine: "Our medical men are becoming a race of carvers," the novelist Elizabeth Stuart Phelps Ward informed members of the Massachusetts legislature in 1901. "Dog or man, cat or baby, it does not matter so much—the fashion is to slice. Human vivisection follows animal vivisection naturally and easily, secretly or openly."[116]

Chapter Two

The Charge of Human Vivisection

 In October 1897 Dr. Albert Tracy Leffingwell warned the delegates to the twenty-first annual convention of the American Humane Association (AHA) that a new threat to the existing moral order had arisen: "the Assassination of Human Beings as a Means of Scientific Research."[1] As he described the "scientific murders" committed by the Italian physician Giuseppe Sanarelli, who had injected five patients with the "bacillus of yellow fever" in a South American hospital, Leffingwell reminded his audience that such experimentation was confined neither to European physicians nor to foreign hospitals. In the past year, he declared, similar experiments had been conducted in public hospitals in Maryland and Massachusetts—investigations performed for reasons other than the benefit of the individual patients, investigations ending, in some cases, in death.

The delegates were disheartened but not surprised by Leffingwell's disclosures. "Having read the accounts of the horrid and cruel destruction of life which has been inflicted upon millions of animals," AHA president John G. Shortall grimly observed, "I have been expecting every year to hear of the experimenter reaching man."[2] At the close of the meeting, the AHA adopted a resolution condemning Sanarelli's scientific murders and appointing Leffingwell to a committee to study the practice of experimenting on human beings.

Why did the American Humane Association, an organization primarily devoted to animal protection, launch an effort to protect human beings from experimentation by doctors? Historians of the American animal protection and antivivisection movements have paid little attention to the issue of human vivisection.[3] I argue that American opposition to animal experimentation cannot be understood independently of the expectation, shared by most antivivisectionists and many animal protectionists, that unrestrained experimentation on animals would culminate in the scientific exploitation of vulnerable human beings. Although the animal protection and antivivisection societies parted company (around 1910) over the best methods to achieve their goals, the charge of human vivisection continued to play a salient role in antivivisectionist critiques of unrestricted animal experimentation during the first four decades of the twentieth century. To understand how the issue of human vivisection came to be so closely identified with protecting animals, we need to examine the development of the animal protection and antivivisection movements in the second half of the nineteenth century.

Before 1866, concern about animal welfare was almost exclusively a private matter. To be sure, some state legislatures had before the Civil War enacted statutes prohibiting cruelty to animals, but there is little evidence that such laws were either enforced or even well known.[4] Henry Bergh (1823–88) changed all this. Serving in the American diplomatic corps in St. Petersburg, Russia, Bergh had been troubled by the mistreatment of carriage horses. His interest in animal protection intensified after a visit to London, where he attended several meetings of the Royal Society for the Prevention of Cruelty to Animals (founded in 1824). After his return to New York, Bergh dedicated himself to creating an American animal protection society. With the support of several wealthy New Yorkers (including John Jacob Astor, who made his fortune in the fur trade), Bergh established the American Society for the Prevention of Cruelty to Animals (ASPCA) in 1866.[5]

The ASPCA provided a model for humane advocates in other cities. In 1867, Caroline Earle White, with the support of Bergh and the city's social elite, organized the Pennsylvania Society for the Prevention of Cruelty to Animals (PSPCA), in Philadelphia. The following year prosperous attorney George T. Angell drafted the act of incorporation for the Massachusetts Society for the Prevention of Cruelty to Animals, in Boston. Similar organizations were soon founded in New Jersey, San Francisco, Illinois, and Minnesota.[6]

In the 1870s humane organizations expanded their anticruelty focus to include children. Although Bergh initially resisted child protection, arguing that other charitable organizations cared for children, he continued to receive both appeals from individuals seeking aid for abused and neglected children and criticism from newspapers about his apparent preference for animals.[7] In 1874 the case of Mary Ellen Wilson, a 9-year-old girl beaten by her stepmother, roused Bergh's interest in child protection. After the prosecution of Mary Ellen's stepmother, Bergh, together with his attorney, Elbridge T. Gerry, and John D. Wright, a wealthy Quaker, organized the New York Society for the Prevention of Cruelty to Children (incorporated in 1875). The ASPCA and the SPCC worked closely together; Gerry served as counsel to both groups. (Today visitors to the ASPCA offices in New York City can view the scissors Mary Ellen's stepmother used to punish the young girl.)[8] In large cities like Boston, where the Massachusetts Society for the Prevention of Cruelty to Children was founded in 1878, humane advocates established separate organizations to pursue child protection.[9] In many smaller cities humane organizations performed the dual functions of animal and child protection. Reasons of efficiency and the demands of fundraising encouraged some separation of child protection from animal protection. Other groups insisted that the two were naturally linked. "The protection of children and the protection of animals," argued the Colorado Bureau of Child and Animal Protection, "are combined because of the principle involved, i.e. their helplessness, is the same; because all life is the same, differing only in degree of development and expression; and because each profits by association with the other."[10]

The last two decades of the nineteenth century saw rapid growth in the number of animal and child protection societies across the country. In order to coordinate the activities of local humane societies, animal and child protectionists in 1874 created a national organization, the American Humane Association. By 1909 the AHA was reporting that of the 334 societies actively working to prevent cruelty in the United States, 104 organizations were devoting their efforts exclusively to animals, 45 to children, and the remaining 185 to both animal and child protection. These organizations in 1909 boasted a yearly income from endowments and other sources of more than 1.2 million dollars, reported more than 35,000 prosecutions involving cruelty, and involved an estimated 42 million people in their combined activities.[11]

Why did large numbers of Americans join humane societies in the last quarter of the nineteenth century? "Kindness to animals," argues historian James C. Turner, "profaned no social taboos and upset no economic applecarts, either in the theoretical systems of political economists or in the harsh daily encounter of capital and labor."[12] In addition to providing a nonthreatening outlet for the middle-class men and women who joined humane societies, Turner maintains, organized animal protection reflected the wider acceptance of human and animal kinship fostered by Darwinism as well as a desire to modify or reform the work habits and leisure activities of the poor and immigrants and "a general psychological reaction to modernization," creating a longing for some realignment with the natural world.[13]

Kindness to animals and the activities of various humane societies may also have ameliorated the increasingly harsh conditions of urban animal life in the second half of the nineteenth century. Although subjected to ridicule for their efforts, Henry Bergh and his colleagues believed that the ten drinking fountains financed and constructed by the ASPCA in New York City made a difference in the daily lives of urban animals. When Bergh stationed a person to count the number of patrons at one urban fountain, he found that, during a three-hour period on an August day in 1867, 10 dogs, 80 horses, and 850 men, women, and children used the fountain.[14] In addition to providing water and care for injured animals, Bergh pushed for restrictions on the practice of overloading horses. Limiting the number of persons in a street car to a certain number was not a trivial action. Nearly forty thousand horses died in New York City alone between 1880 and 1885, and the worsening conditions for urban animals was a real, not symbolic, concern for animal protectionists.[15]

Henry Bergh initially devoted most of his energies to the protection of horses, pet animals, and livestock (especially transport of cattle by rail). His attention quickly turned to uncovering cruelties in a more novel setting than city streets—to medical institutions in which animals were used for research and teaching. First introduced into American medical education in the 1850s, vivisectional demonstrations became a routine feature of physiology teaching in New York medical schools after the Civil War.[16] Although medical students had occasionally used animals, and even themselves, in physiological researches since the late eighteenth century, the establishment of physiological laboratories at Harvard and Johns Hopkins in the 1870s signaled a new stage of American medical education, attracting the notice of animal protectionists.[17]

Bergh launched the first offensive against cruelty to animals in medical institutions. In public assemblies and in the press, he assailed the vivisection of animals as the "most fearful and revolting" practice "of all the horrible pangs inflicted upon the animal creation."[18] In 1866, the same year he established the ASPCA, he demanded an investigation of cruel laboratory practices at the College of Physicians and Surgeons in New York City, and there first encountered John Call Dalton, one of a pioneering generation of American physiologists.

Dalton's interest in vivisectional demonstrations dated from his own experiences in the laboratory of Claude Bernard. Inspired by the pathbreaking experiments of the French physiologist, Dalton attempted to recreate Bernard's teachings in the lectures he delivered to medical students after his return to New York in the 1850s. He repeated many of the investigations he had witnessed in Bernard's laboratory, including demonstrations on dogs of the action of pancreatic juice and the production of sugar in the liver. Dalton also duplicated Pierre Flourens's experiments on pigeons; his medical students observed that the birds, following removal of selected sections of the brain, survived the procedure even though they lacked the ability to form mental associations.[19]

Similar experiments on pigeons at another New York medical school prompted an investigation by Bergh and agents of the ASPCA. In 1867 a letter from an anonymous student at the Bellevue Hospital Medical College asked Bergh to look into the "wanton cruelty" of physiologist Austin Flint, Jr. "To many of his experiments on dogs and cats under the influence of ether, one can take no exception," the student confided. However, Flint's failure to use ether when opening the head of a pigeon and extracting a portion of the brain was more problematic. In seeking the ASPCA's help, the student explained, he "would not be understood as wishing Professor Flint to dispense with a single experiment, but merely to perform them in the least cruel manner."[20] Flint rejected Bergh's suggestion that familiarity with the sight of pain and suffering had robbed him of sensibility, but he invited the animal protectionist to call on him at the medical college and to witness for himself the demonstrations involving animals. Fortunately, humane inspectors in 1868 found little evidence that experimenters, including Flint, had failed to use ether and chloroform in animal experiments.[21]

Bergh's continuing campaign against vivisection inspired Dalton to offer a spirited defense of the chief method of the new physiology. In order to enlist the support of the New York medical profession, including many unfamiliar with vivisection, he outlined the clinical benefits from animal experimentation. "Every important discovery in physiology," he claimed in 1869, "was the direct result of experiments on animals."[22] The discovery of the circulation of the blood, the processes of respiration, and the function of the spinal nerves, Dalton explained, all had resulted from animal experimentation. His list of the therapeutic advances from experiments on animals was much less impressive. He cited the Hunterian operation for repair of aneurism, blood transfusion (seldom performed before the discovery of blood groups in 1900), and the proper method of administering treatment for venomous snake bites.[23]

Dalton's defense of animal experimentation failed to convert the ASPCA president. Committed to the abolition of all experiments on living animals, Bergh initially attempted to include a clause prohibiting animal vivisection in a cruelty to animals bill before the state legislature in 1867. After the British Parliament enacted the Cruelty to Animals Act in 1876, which placed severe restrictions on animal experimenters in Great Britain, Bergh once again attempted to criminalize vivisection. In 1880 he pressed for legislation to prohibit the practice of vivisection in New York, without success. The New York medical societies condemned his actions, and medical associations across the nation added their disapproval of the proposed restrictions on experimental medicine.[24]

During his lifetime, Bergh dominated the organization he had established. The ASPCA was both an animal protection and antivivisection organization, reflecting Bergh's intense suspicion of experimenting doctors. After his death in 1888, the organization began to retreat from Bergh's hardline views about animal experimentation. Other humane organizations also experienced tensions between animal protection and antivivisection objectives and over the strategies to achieve these goals. At the 1892 meeting of the American Humane Association, for example, delegates approved by a vote of 24 to 19 a resolution calling on state legislatures to adopt laws that prohibited painful experiments on animals for the sole purpose of demonstrating well-known facts. Many of the delegates who opposed the measure were unhappy that the resolution did not go further. They demanded the abolition of painful experimentation on animals.[25]

The failure of mainstream animal protection organizations, like the ASPCA, to continue to condemn vivisection promoted the formation of exclusively antivivisectionist groups. The first such organization, the American Anti-Vivisection Society, was established in Philadelphia in 1883 by Caroline Earle White, one of the founders of the Pennsylvania SPCA.[26] The changes in the name of White's organization during the first four years of its existence reflected some of the tensions between animal protection and antivivisection, as well as differences over immediatist and gradualist approaches to the problem of animal experimentation. In 1883 members of the group voted to change the name of the association to the American Society for the Restriction of Vivisection. In 1887, they returned to the original name.[27] White, who served as editor of the group's monthly magazine, the *Journal of Zoophily*, until her death in 1916, remained a lifelong proponent of the total abolition of animal experimentation.

In other cities, critics of animal experimentation also organized societies: in Boston, the New England Anti-Vivisection Society (1895); in New York, the Society for Prevention of Abuse in Animal Experimentation (1907), the New York Anti-Vivisection Society (1908), and the Vivisection Investigation League (1912); in Baltimore, the Anti-Vivisection Society of Maryland (1898); and in Illinois, the Vivisection Reform Society (1903 in Chicago) and the Illinois Anti-Vivisection Society (1892 in Aurora). In California several antivivisectionist societies joined forces to create the California Federation of Anti-Vivisection Societies (1918), representing groups from Los Angeles, San Francisco, and Alameda County. Antivivisectionist groups in Washington State and Colorado also campaigned for restrictions on vivisection.[28]

The focus on laboratory animals of these newly organized antivivisection societies did not diminish their investment in general animal protection. In fact, antivivisection and animal protection continued to overlap in significant ways. In addition to her efforts on behalf of laboratory animals, Caroline White organized a temporary pound to house stray and homeless small animals collected from city streets. Aided by a grant of $2500 from the city of Philadelphia, her organization assumed responsibility for these animals.[29]

American antivivisectionists devoted considerable energy to the welfare of cattle and horses. In the 1870s and 1880s, when investigations by humane society agents revealed that cattle were routinely shipped in closely packed railway cars without food or water for as much as 72 hours, antivivisectionists and animal protectionists appealed to Congress for protective laws. The Women's Branch of the PSPCA subsequently brought charges against the Reading Railroad for violating laws protecting cattle during transport.[30] In 1907 White was instrumental in obtaining a congressional investigation of railroad animal transportation, which resulted in a federal law compelling companies to feed and water animals in their care at least once every twenty-eight hours. She often characterized this law as the "crowning achievement" of her life.[31] When several entrepreneurs attempted to import and popularize the Spanish style of bull fighting in the United States, antivivisectionists added their voices against the practice.[32] They also sponsored the construction of water troughs for horses and helped to maintain ambulances and hospitals for injured and rescued animals.[33]

White actively campaigned against the use of birds or any part of their plumage in women's attire. At the beginning of the twentieth century, bird protectionists claimed that more than 200 million birds were killed every year for their feathers, and the methods of plume hunters produced a dramatic decline in the populations of sea, shore, and marsh birds. In addition to serving as honorary vice presidents of the Audubon Society, White and her co-workers attempted to enlist support from members of the Woman's Christian Temperance Union (WCTU) for their "Appeal to Women Not to Wear Birds or Their Plumage."[34] In 1913 the actress and antivivisectionist Minnie Maddern Fiske, who aided Diana Belais's founding of the New York Anti-Vivisection Society, organized a boycott of milliners who sold aigrette plumes.[35] Cruelties in the fur trade also concerned antivivisectionists. "The principal device used by professional trappers," Caroline White advised women, "is the steel trap, the most villainous instrument of arrest that was ever invented by the human mind."[36] In addition to the cruel specter of a captured animal attempting to gnaw off a leg in order to escape, antivivisectionists invoked the damaging effects on young men and boys of trapping animals. The commitment to animal protection outside the laboratory persisted in the first half of the twentieth century. In a continuing effort to wean women from cruelty in dress, the American Anti-Vivisection Society in the 1920s sponsored a humane alternative to animal skins, a synthetic fur substitute called "humanifur." When a delegation from the fur industry donated a fur coat to the President's wife in 1925, Minnie Fiske successfully persuaded Mrs. Calvin Coolidge not to wear the offending garment.[37]

The American antivivisectionist movement, as is suggested by the varying names of the organizations (and the strains within White's own Philadelphia society over restriction versus abolition), encompassed a spectrum of opinions about animal experimentation and the means by which reform could be achieved. Whereas the goal pursued by White and her associates was nothing short of the elimination of vivisection, other groups and individuals adopted a less extreme position. They favored restrictions on animal experimentation or vivisection reform, rather than total opposition to vivisection, arguing that animal experimentation was acceptable if legal safeguards were in place to insure the welfare of laboratory animals.

The reform position deserves serious consideration. A survey conducted by the American Humane Association in 1895 suggested widespread support for a moderate stance on vivisection. When the AHA polled 2,086 members of "the more educated classes of the United States," 1,753 (84.1%)

of the clergymen, educators, writers, editors, and doctors opposed unlimited animal experimentation. Only 281 (13.4%) favored vivisection without restrictions on the use of anesthetics or purpose.

Like the other professional groups polled by the AHA, most physicians endorsed some regulation of vivisection. Of the 1,239 physicians in New York and Massachusetts who participated, only 220 (19.1%) opposed any legal restriction of vivisection. However, nearly the same number, 207 (18%), urged a total prohibition of experiments on animals.[38] The majority favored "reasonable restrictions" on animal experimentation. These physicians hardly represented a random sample of doctors, since most had practiced medicine for at least fifteen years. As older physicians, they may have been less likely to have witnessed vivisectional demonstrations during their medical training. But, even some graduates of more advanced medical schools advocated restrictions on vivisection. "It appears to me," noted Harvard Medical School alumnus Albert H. Blanchard, "that the advantages of vivisection, and the practical good derived therefrom are not, at present, sufficient to justify its practice unless it can be done without pain."[39]

Critics of antivivisection tended to ignore this moderate stance, arguing that all attempts at reform were merely "the entering wedge" for legislation forbidding the practice of animal experimentation.[40] Some medical observers, however, acknowledged the sincerity of reform motives. "Conservative anti-vivisection," noted the writer of an 1896 editorial in the *Medical Record*, "is a legitimate agitation."[41] Roswell McCrea, an early historian of the humane movement and no friend of antivivisection, named the Vivisection Reform Society as an example of an organization apparently sincere in the effort to combat abuses of vivisection without necessarily abolishing the practice.[42]

Few records from antivivisectionist societies have survived, and information about the women and men who joined is generally difficult to obtain.[43] From the first, one of the distinctive features of these organizations was their overwhelmingly female identity. Although men appeared prominently on boards of directors and lists of honorary vice presidents, women outnumbered men in the membership rolls, and they provided much of the financial support for the organizations. The activities of the New York–based Society for the Prevention of Abuse in Animal Experimentation was made possible by a generous female backer. Women also bequeathed 41 of the 44 legacies (ranging in value from $25 to $10,200) received by the New England Anti-Vivisection Society in the years 1898 to

1935. Perhaps not surprisingly, the three estates left by men were considerably larger; the NEAVS received $19,807, $25,000, and $30,231 from male donors.[44]

Women assumed positions of leadership in the antivivisection and animal protection movements. At the American Anti-Vivisection Society, Caroline Earle White was joined by Adele Biddle, the daughter of a prominent Philadelphia family, and by Mary S. Lovell. Lovell provided crucial support for the antivivisection cause in her capacity as the national superintendent of the Department of Mercy of the Woman's Christian Temperance Union, the largest women's organization in the country. In New York Diana Belais founded and guided as president the New York Anti-Vivisection Society. When tension within Belais's organization arose, two prominent women, Sue M. Farrell and her niece Maud Ingersoll Probasco, resigned and established a second New York organization, the Vivisection Investigation League. Women also played an active role in the California and Chicago antivivisection societies.

The prominence of women in the antivivisection movement and their frequent appeals to sentiment provided a handy target for their critics. Medical observers acidly noted the spectacle of large numbers of women attending antivivisectionist meetings wearing furs or "murderous millinery," hats adorned with feathers or even entire birds. Others warned of the potential menace of granting voting rights to such women, who might be ruled by "wild gusts of unreasoning, uncalculating, hysterical emotion."[45] Even the American feminist Elizabeth Cady Stanton counted "the hysterical force in favor of prohibition, a Puritan Sabbath, antivivisection, and religion in the United States Constitution" among the reasons for male hesitation in giving women the ballot.[46]

Speculation by physicians about the women who swelled the ranks of antivivisection societies proved remarkably persistent. Like New York neurologist Charles Dana, Dr. James Warbasse identifed investment in antivivisection as a special form of female psychopathology. Warbasse advised readers in 1910 that an exaggerated sympathy for dogs on the part of women was a manifestation of a "zoophilic psychosis."[47] Rather than interest themselves in the welfare of mice, snakes, cattle, chicken, and sheep, Warbasse insisted, women doted "on those useless animals which can be made the objects of fondling and which compared with other animals play a minor role in the great field of scientific experimentation." Noting that a German physician had divided women into two types, "the mother class and the prostitute-type," Warbasse asserted that women with an attachment for dogs did not belong to the "mother type."[48]

The women who joined antivivisectionist societies discounted such observations; they valued the moral and emotional commitments that had led to their involvement in animal protection. They celebrated the feminine emotions of love and compassion that fueled their opposition to animal experimentation, even as their sentiments were being disparaged by male critics. Female physicians helped lead the charge. When the surgeon William W. Keen dismissed the antivivisection movement as "a lot of zoophilist women," Dr. Amanda M. Hale, employed as a lecturer by the American Anti-Vivisection Society, insisted that zoophilist women needed no apology. Men, Hale argued, were "egotists. Not realizing that woman's affections are as broad and deep as the boundless seas, they are not willing that even a little wavelet shall overflow upon poor Fido or Prince. They want it all for themselves."[49] Rather than standing in the way of the world's progress, Hale insisted, women like Frances Willard, president of the WCTU, and physicians Josephine Butler and Elizabeth Blackwell were leading the rescue of the human race from "social perdition."

Rescuing the human race was precisely the agenda that Elizabeth Blackwell, the first female graduate of an American medical school, set for herself when she decided on a medical career. Although she emigrated to England soon after setting up the Women's Medical College of the New York Infirmary in 1869, Blackwell remained an important role model for antivivisectionist physicians like Amanda Hale. An outspoken critic of animal experimentation throughout her professional life, Blackwell emphasized the unique moral sensibility that women brought to medicine. "Bacteriology and its penchant for vaccination offended Blackwell," argues historian Regina Morantz Sanchez, "because its concept of specific etiology undermined her sense of the moral order. A concomitant of modern laboratory science—animal experimentation—represented something much worse."[50] Blackwell correlated the increase in sexual surgery on women in the late nineteenth century with the spread of animal experimentation, warning that the reckless sacrifice of animal life "tends to make us less scrupulous in our treatment of the sick and helpless poor. It increases that disposition to regard the poor as 'clinical material,' which has become, alas! not without reason, a widespread approach to many of the young members of our most honourable and merciful profession."[51] When the Women's Medical College established an experimental laboratory in 1891, Blackwell sent a letter protesting this unfortunate development and the necessary hardening it would entail.[52] Many antivivisectionists shared Blackwell's belief in the higher moral sense of women, her desire to restore moral sensibility to medicine, and her rejection of the new medical sciences.

The relationship Blackwell identified between animal experimentation and sexual surgery on women has been invoked to explain the recruitment of women into the British antivivisection movement. Coral Lansbury has argued that in Victorian England women embraced antivivisection not simply for humanitarian reasons "but because the vivisected animal stood for vivisected woman: the woman strapped to the gynaecologist's table, the woman strapped and bound in the pornographic fiction of the period."[53] In a more nuanced study, Mary Ann Elston identified "the metaphor of medical science, and medical practice on women, as rape" as a dominant theme in British antivivisection literature after 1880.[54]

These motifs played a less salient role in the American antivivisection movement. Sexual surgery and the "vivisection of women" never received as much attention in the American literature as they did from British antivivisectionists. The theme of sexual victimization was not entirely absent from the American scene. The identification of women with vivisected animals and the sexual sadism of male vivisectors was intimated in the two antivivisectionist novels of the popular author Elizabeth Stuart Phelps (later Ward). In *Trixy* (1904) and *Though Life Us Do Part* (1908), Phelps suggested that men treated women like pets: "A man may vivisect a woman nerve by nerve, anguish by anguish."[55] Most American antivivisectionists, however, placed greater emphasis on special female responsibilities for guiding moral development than on the rhetoric of rape.

Female antivivisectionists embraced a duty to inculcate kindness and compassion for the helpless—animal and human. Although dismissed by some medical critics as "unmarried or sterile old women whose maternal affections are centered on animals instead of babies," female antivivisectionists privileged the responsibility for molding young minds and developing compassion and kindness for humans and animals alike.[56] The massive investment in humane education and "juvenile work" illustrated their commitment to guiding the moral development of the young, as well as the important links between the temperance movement and organized antivivisection.

The Women's Branch of the Pennsylvania SPCA, led by Caroline White and Mary Lovell, formally began the educational mission for children. In 1874 they organized Junior Humane Societies to train boys in the ways of kindness.[57] Although George T. Angell and other male leaders of the animal protection movement also developed programs for humane education, Lovell argued that systematic humane education could best be conducted by women, because women had the time and resources to devote themselves to it over a long period.[58] Humane education became Lovell's life work. "Any society for the prevention of cruelty, whether composed of men or women or of both, which neglects humane education is missing its greatest opportunity," she informed delegates of the American Humane Association in 1899.[59]

In 1890 the movement for humane education received a powerful boost when the Woman's Christian Temperance Union formally adopted a department of mercy as one of its divisions, and WCTU president Frances Willard appointed Mary Lovell as national departmental superintendent. Joining other WCTU departments, which included ones for peace, suppression of impure literature, suppression of sabbath desecration, and physical education, Lovell's division embraced work with children.[60] Like her mentor, Mary Hanchett Hunt (the powerful superintendent of the WCTU's Department of Scientific Temperance Instruction), Mary Lovell soon pressed for state laws to establish humane education in public schools. By 1906 Lovell claimed success in the twelve states that had adopted laws prescribing humane education in public schools.[61]

The Department of Mercy also promoted humane education by organizing "bands of mercy," groups of schoolchildren who pledged to be kind to animals. In 1899 Lovell reported that nearly 14,000 boys in public schools in Philadelphia alone were enrolled in Bands of Mercy. By 1923 more than 140,000 bands of mercy in the United States claimed more than 4 million child members.[62]

The bands of mercy had a significant influence on the activities of children in the United States. The Salvation Army, for example, adopted "bands of love," in which children pledged to love animals and to be kind to them. The Boy Scouts, too, adopted kindness to animals as one of the obligations of scouthood.[63] In the second decade of the twentieth century, scouts could aspire to a merit badge in first aid to animals. In order to qualify, not only did scouts have to demonstrate their ability to treat domestic and farm animals, they were also required to know how to aid a horse in harness when it fell on the street and what action to take when animals were being cruelly mistreated.[64]

The level of anticruelty activity varied enormously among these groups. Many children no doubt confined their participation in bands of mercy to taking the pledge to be kind to animals and wearing a membership button. The varying quality of participation, however, should not obscure the ideological commitment on the part of educators, teachers, and humane advocates to the idea that childhood lessons in kindness to animals promised great benefit. Many Americans accepted the association of cruelty to animals in childhood with subsequent sadism and criminality in adulthood; for antivivisectionists this linkage was virtually an article of faith.

Boys in particular were considered in need of instruction and moral teaching. "The average boy will kill [an animal] without thought or regret. This may not be the fault of the boy, but because, perhaps, nature did not give him the tender heart," Mrs. Fairchild-Allen of the Illinois Anti-Vivisection Society observed. Where nature failed, parents and teachers were required "to create a new heart." Statistics from France and America, she argued, demonstrated that a large proportion of the inmates of jails and penitentiaries were never taught kindness to animals and lacked pets during their childhood.[65] Other antivivisectionists likened vivisectors to little boys who never grew up. As children, such boys took delight in breaking their toys; as adults, they dismembered sentient animals with the same mindless glee.[66]

Antivivisectionists accepted responsibility for molding moral conscience, and children represented the most accessible audience for an education in kindness. Female responsibility for inculcating morality, however, extended beyond childhood's edge. Mary Lovell, for example, applied the maternal approach to the conduct of nations. In 1898 she likened the world to a school and Spain's "misrule and barbarous cruelties" in Cuba to a cruel bully exercising tyranny over a weaker pupil.[67] The American rescue of Cuba from the Spanish, Lovell argued, did not represent the best solution. Rather than by armed intervention, the crisis might best have been resolved by "humane statesmen and stateswomen" joining together to cultivate the humane sentiment of nations, to civilize the "semi-developed," and to prevent the carnage of war.

The risk posed to human beings by the demoralizing effect of unrestrained cruelty to animals was not the only argument advanced against unrestricted animal experimentation. Antivivisectionists also disputed the clinical benefits of animal vivisection.[68] Faithful to a traditional paradigm that explained disease as a consequence of filth and putrefaction, many antivivisectionists insisted that medical progress would result from the implementation of conventional methods of sanitary science.[69] In 1899, seventeen years after Robert Koch's identification of the tubercle bacillus, anti-

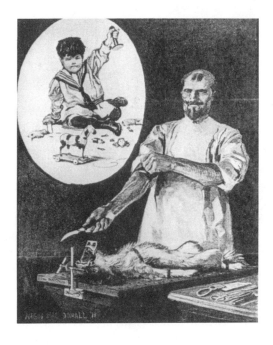

"The Little Boy Who Never Grew Up," antivivisectionist depiction of vivisectors as heartless. *Life*, 1911.

vivisectionist physician Amanda Hale continued to inform audiences that tuberculosis was not contagious. "We must look for the causes of consumption along the old familiar lines," she remarked. Her list of suspect agents included hereditary predisposition, bad food, bad water, and consanguineous marriages.[70] The faddish reliance on animal experimentation, antivivisectionists insisted, was in fact bad science.

Not surprisingly, these same individuals rejected the utility of serums and vaccines and protested their development through bacteriological techniques. There was considerable overlap between the antivaccination and antivivisection causes. Antivivisectionist publications (such as *The Open Door*, edited by Diana Belais, president of the New York Anti-Vivisection Society) routinely published stories critical of vaccination and vaccine therapy involving the injection of diseased animal blood into human tissue. Even antivivisectionists who accepted the germ theory of disease disputed the claims of utility advanced by defenders of unrestricted medical research. Declaring that the discoveries from animal experimentation had been much exaggerated, several antivivisectionists insisted that such medical benefits as the discovery of a treatment to prevent childbed fever, or puerperal sepsis, actually came from clinical experiences rather than laboratory experiments.[71] In light of differences among species, they similarly questioned the clinical value of cerebral localization studies performed on monkeys.[72]

Arguments about the morality of harming sentient creatures for the purposes of enhancing scientific knowledge took precedence over the issue of clinical benefit. Frequently quoted was Jeremy Bentham's dictum about the moral considerability of animals: "The question is not, Can they reason? nor Can they talk? but Can they suffer?"[73] David H. Cochran, former president of the Brooklyn Polytechnic, echoed this sentiment: "The endowment of sensibility is the endowment of rights. Without sensibility there is no right. A being without sensibility can suffer no wrong."[74] No progress in medicine, many antivivisectionists argued, was worth the pain inflicted in laboratories by physicians and physiologists. Most animal protectionists refused to accept the stark formulations of such active campaigners for the freedom of research as Charles W. Eliot, president of Harvard University. "How many cats, or guinea pigs," Eliot frequently asked, "would you or I sacrifice to save the life of our child, or to win the chance of saving the life of our child?"[75] John Ames Mitchell, the editor of *Life* magazine, sarcastically retorted that some people might be willing to sacrifice a few college presidents, but even desperation wouldn't make it morally right. Mitchell instead compared the emotionally charged child-or-guinea-pig appeal to the old antiabolitionist cry: "Do you want your daughter to marry a Negro?"[76]

A preoccupation with pain and suffering in the laboratory marked antivivisectionist periodicals, whose pages were filled with graphic descriptions of animals undergoing various techniques for the purposes of experimentation. Perhaps more compelling were illustrations and photographs of animals in actual vivisectional apparatus. Some antivivisection organizations rented storefronts in busy commercial districts and exhibited stuffed animals in vivisectional apparatus. The American Anti-Vivisection Society, for example, developed an exhibit, which traveled in major cities, including New York, Boston, Philadelphia, Los Angeles, and Baltimore.[77]

Images of antivivisectional apparatus also reached the public through the popular weekly *Life*, which in 1890 claimed a circulation of 50,000 readers. *Life* functioned as an unofficial organ of antivivisectionist and antivaccinationist sentiment, reflecting the views of the magazine's founder and editor, John Mitchell.[78] Mitchell's reliance on comic vignettes about vivisecting doctors (Drs. Slasher Quick and Futyll Werk, and Catcarver Jones, M.D.) and cartoons depicting "the animals' revenge" (dogs experimenting on a vivisector) and "the short step" (the vivisector's short walk from the experimental laboratory to the hospital ward) led one hostile reader to suggest that Mitchell should have renamed the magazine *Death*.[79]

Antivivisectionists were not the only Americans preoccupied with pain. The discovery of anesthesia in the 1840s, which greatly advanced the use of vivisectional techniques by minimizing animal distress (and the concomitant distress of the experimenter), made painful procedures in the absence of anesthesia seem more horrible. In part, this explained the repugnance with which antivivisectionists regarded François Magendie, also known as the Arch-Fiend, whose animal experiments were largely performed before anesthesia was available. Increased sensitivity to suffering did not escape nineteenth-century observers.[80] "We no longer think that we are called upon to face physical pain with equanimity," Harvard psychologist and philosopher William James observed in 1902, contending that the changing attitude toward pain constituted a watershed in modern sensibility. "It is not expected of a man that he should either endure it or inflict much of it," James argued, "and to listen to the recitals of cases of it makes our flesh creep morally as well as physically."[81]

Presumably, physicians and physiologists were not unaffected by the new sensitivity to pain. Although recently sociologists have identified the use of "gallows" humor as a means to relieve some of the anxieties associated with autopsy and experimentation on live animals, nineteenth-century antivivisectionists construed medical school pranks and buffoonery quite differently.[82] Stories about medical students "ball-playing with corpses" and reports of students sewing two puppies together appeared in antivivisectionist literature as evidence of the demoralization that dissection and vivisection necessarily entailed.[83]

That the practice of vivisection, the deliberate and calculated infliction of pain in the name of medical science, diminished sensitivity to suffering most antivivisectionists accepted without question. Cleland Kinloch Nelson, an Atlanta clergyman, echoed popular sentiment among antivivisectionists when he wrote: "Were I on the bench I should never admit as either juror or witness in a criminal case any one who practiced vivisection or regularly attended lectures on the subject. I am convinced that the tendency of these exploits is to blunt the finer instincts of our nature, to harden people to the cries of pain."[84]

The notion that cruelty to animals blunted ethical sensibilities was not born in the nineteenth century. Both classical moralists and medieval scholastics condemned cruelty to animals because of its brutalizing effect on human character. In the seventeenth and eighteenth centuries, butchers were regarded with misgivings for similar reasons. Slaughterhouse workers endured suspicion "not just because of the noise, smell, blood and pollution which their activities involved, but also because of a widespread aversion to the act of slaughter itself."[85] At least some suspicion that butchering adversely affected moral sensibility persisted into the nineteenth century. Amid the panic occasioned by the murders associated with Jack the Ripper, one London minister recommended that all slaughterhouses in the district be closed down as part of a preventive program.[86] American antivivisectionists pointed to a nineteenth-century Pennsylvania law that forbade butchers to serve on juries deciding capital offenses, and they warned that, like butchers, surgeons were liable to lose the finer instincts.[87] Often quoted was Alfred Lord Tennyson's line about the surgeon who "was happier using the knife than in trying to save the limb."[88] Belief in the occupational hazards of surgery led some antivivisectionists to correlate an apparent increase in the murders committed by medical students and physicians with the rise of vivisection.[89]

Closely related to distrust of experimenting physicians was public disquiet about autopsy. Public suspicion of physicians' "mangling the dead to satisfy an idle curiosity" led D. W. Cathell, author of a popular text on professional success in medicine, to advise circumspection in persuading families to allow postmortem dissections.[90] Opposition to dissection, of course, has an ancient history. In late nineteenth-century America, continuing public resistance to dissection created chronic shortages of bodies for use in medical education.[91] Although by 1915 anatomy acts in many states had increased the supply of legal cadavers, continuing shortages created a clandestine traffic in corpses, which included interstate shipment of black bodies to northern medical schools.[92] Stories in the popular press about grave-robbing incidents and conspiracies to provide newly dead paupers for medical school autopsies fed public fears about "dissecting doctors."[93]

Antivivisectionists introduced another fear: that dissection or autopsy could begin on living individuals. Concern that doctors were not always able to make a positive determination of death prompted some antivivisectionists to support the popular, if short-lived, Society for the Prevention of Premature Burial.[94] Insisting that decay was the only sure sign of death, George T. Angell, founder of the Massachusetts Society for the Prevention of Cruelty to Animals, petitioned the United States Congress in 1896 to require "a careful and competent inspection, *previous to* burial, of all persons *supposed* to be dead."[95] Although physicians, not unnaturally, resented the suggestion that their professional incompetence led to the premature burial of the supposed dead, the dread of premature burial reportedly led such notables as Herbert Spencer, Benjamin Ward Richardson, Hans Christian Andersen, and Wilkie Collins to leave written instructions in their will to the effect that after their apparent death the physician would pierce their heart with a needle or sever the carotid artery, as a guarantee that life was extinct.[96] In accordance with her instructions, when the well-known English antivivisectionist Frances Power Cobbe died in 1903, a telegram was sent to a colleague of hers, physician Walter Hadwen, who obliged by severing the carotid artery of the body, "in order to ensure that she was really dead."[97]

Mutual emphases on powerlessness and pain marked the rhetoric of the movement against premature burial and vivisection. Like the descriptions of animals confined in the vivisector's laboratory, the narratives of being buried alive stressed the victim's panic, claustrophobia, and anguished struggles for freedom.

In the case of animal experimentation, of course, the root cause of suffering was not a physician's inability to determine death but his scientific ambition. Suspicion of the overzealous pursuit of scientific knowledge is evident in a quotation that appeared ubiquitously in antivivisection literature, a sentence culled from an article written by E. E. Slosson, a University of Wyoming chemist, that appeared in a religious newspaper in 1895: "A human life is nothing compared to a new fact in science."[98] Slosson never practiced vivisection and was in fact referring to autoexperimentation by researchers, but he was nonetheless cited as an example *par excellence* of the willingness of medical researchers to sacrifice anything or anyone in order to assuage scientific curiosity. Antivivisectionists warned repeatedly that the failure to enact legislative safeguards for animal subjects would inevitably lead to human experimentation.

Medical proposals to vivisect criminals condemned to death intensified antivivisectionist concerns. In 1893 an Ohio physician, John S. Pyle, garnered notoriety for proposing to the Tri-State Medical Society that vivisection of condemned criminals be legalized.[99] In response to the debate over capital punishment and to ongoing concerns that the final punishment be accomplished with as little suffering as possible, Pyle proposed that condemned criminals be enlisted in an ambitious research program to probe the secrets of the human brain and human consciousness:

To secure cooperation and carry out the experiment successfully the condemned would be instructed with the nature of the work, assured that no torture would be instituted; that the preparations of removing a piece of the skull and cerebral membranes should take place when under the influence of an anesthetic; and while he would be allowed to regain consciousness to be interrogated, that no pain should be occasioned thereby; lastly that his death should occur when in a profound sleep.[100]

In Pyle's opinion, this reformed system of punishment not only would rob the process of the spirit of revenge and barbarity, it would also encourage the study of cerebral localization and brain surgery, hampered in the past by lack of access to human brains. Questions about the ethics of using human beings in this manner troubled Pyle very little. He argued that if emotional objections to the use of human subjects in experimental work were raised, it would be incumbent upon critics to prove that there was no right to inflict death as a punishment. Since the State sanctioned the execution of convicted criminals, there could be little or no objection to conducting that policy in a manner consonant with scientific inquiry.[101] Pyle's proposal for the vivisection of criminals was introduced into the Ohio legislature in 1894 but, despite the support of several clergymen, physicians, and lawyers, did not pass the General Assembly.[102]

The Ohio proposal received the most attention, but it was not the only call in support of the vivisection of criminals condemned to death. In 1903 the *Journal of Zoophily* reported attempts in Indiana to obtain criminals for scientific experiments. William B. Fletcher of the Central Indiana Hospital for the Insane apparently told newspaper reporters in 1903, "My first thought . . . was to raise funds to purchase in China or any other such market such criminals as were condemned to capital punishment, but there were so many stumbling blocks in the way—the expense, for instance, the lack of physiological and chemical laboratories, lack of knowledge of so-called heathen language, etc."[103] Nor was Fletcher the first to suggest that subjects be purchased. New York newspapers in the 1890s carried advertisements offering compensation to individuals willing to become subjects of medical experiments.[104] Before the Civil War some southern physicians had actually used slaves as experimental subjects, advertising from time to time their wish to purchase Negroes with particular complaints in order to test new remedies.[105]

Antivivisectionists greeted the proposals of Pyle and Fletcher with alarm. Mary Lovell regarded them in apocalyptic terms, as "the fulfillment of prophecy" about the insatiable and remorseless curiosity of physiologists, whose appetites for experimentation had been whetted rather than appeased by unrestricted animal experimentation. "To those who know the long history of starving, burning, scalding, freezing, flaying, injecting irritants into intestines and into eye-balls, tearing out nerves, putting virus into brain, and all the other numerous devices of the experimenter," Lovell declared, the promises of painless experimentation made by prospective human vivisectors were "a ridiculous as well as terrible mockery."[106]

Defenders of animal experimentation argued that human experimentation —on criminals and others—would be the inevitable result of antivivisection-ist interference in medical research. William Williams Keen, then a lecturer in anatomy at the Women's Medical College in Philadelphia, informed the graduating class in 1885: "To grow better we must try new methods, give new drugs, perform new operations, or perform old ones in new ways. That is to say we must experiment. . . . They must then be tried either on an animal or on you. Which shall it be?"[107] Howard A. Kelly, professor of gynecology at Johns Hopkins University School of Medicine, similarly warned of the results of restricting animal experimentation: "If experiments are not made upon animals, then they will be made upon human beings, either, first by the observation of the slow progress of disease, or second, by the entire rising generation of surgeons in gaining that degree of technical skill which their predecessors have obtained."[108] Research advocates were seeking to impress upon the public their urgent need for unrestricted access to animals for medical research. They were *not* promoting human experimentation. Nevertheless, their statements were cited as additional evidence for the inevitability of human vivisection.

As the nineteenth century drew to a close, the issue of human vivisection smoldered within the American antivivisectionist movement. The revelation of Sanarelli's experiments with yellow fever in 1897 kindled Albert Tracy Leffingwell's interest, leading him to thrust the ethical problems posed by research with human subjects into the forefront of American agitation over animal experimentation. Sympathy for the underdog (so to speak) shaped Leffingwell's career as a humane advocate. Born in New York in 1845, Leffingwell studied medicine at the Long Island College Hospital, receiving his medical degree in 1874. Like many young physicians, he traveled abroad to supplement his medical education, attending clinics in Vienna, Paris, and London, where he became interested in the case of a young English girl sentenced to death for destroying her unborn child in her own unsuccessful suicide attempt. Leffingwell's petitions on her behalf helped to convince the British government to commute her death sentence to one year's imprisonment.[109]

Upon his return to New York, Leffingwell joined his uncle James Caleb Jackson and other family members in the administration of the Dansville Sanitarium. Jackson's water cure establishment, whose patrons included

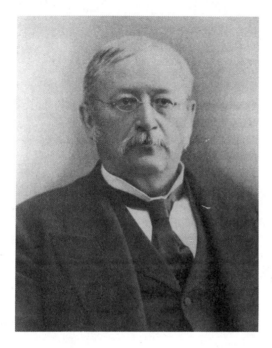

Physician and vivisection reformer Albert T. Leffingwell, M.D. From a report of the American Humane Association, 1906.

Elizabeth Cady Stanton, Susan B. Anthony, Frances E. Willard, and Frederick Douglass, embraced a broad spectrum of nineteenth-century causes: temperance, women's rights, dress reform, and vegetarianism.[110] The financial success of the institution and his marriage to Dr. Elizabeth Fear, a "female practitioner of medicine with considerable ready cash," enabled Leffingwell to relinquish his medical practice and pursue his own reform interests.[111] He began writing for popular periodicals on such topics as illegitimacy, suicide, free trade, pure food, and vivisection.[112]

Beginning in 1880 and continuing until his death in 1916, Leffingwell devoted his energies to vivisection reform. Throughout three decades of agitation for restrictions on animal experimentation, he identified himself as a vivisection reformer, rather than an antivivisectionist. Indeed, he secured an apology from one medical editor who mislabeled him an antivivisectionist. Legal restrictions on experiments on animals, Leffingwell argued, would reduce animal suffering in the laboratory but still allow medical progress to continue.[113] His medical training and his moderate stance as a vivisection reformer conferred on him considerable authority which more strident—and female—antivivisectionists lacked. In 1897 Leffingwell directed his formidable energies and lent his considerable stature to the struggle against using human subjects in medical research.

He first learned of Sanarelli's experiments with yellow fever from a newspaper account. Concern turned to alarm when he read the brisk account by a Washington correspondent who intimated that "unscientific persons" might be "disposed to criticize" such research. In a letter to the editor of the Boston *Transcript*, Leffingwell challenged the claim that only nonscientists might find such reports disturbing: "Does this imply that scientific persons are not so inclined? Must condemnation of such deeds be relegated to the despised class of 'unscientific persons?'"[114]

The experiments with yellow fever and their reception must be seen in the context of medical research on infectious diseases in the late nineteenth century. Control of yellow fever was of obvious importance to the Western nations bent on territorial expansion in the tropics. The Spanish-American War and the acquisition of Cuba and the Philippines lent new urgency to American involvement in the search for ways to control the disease. The pursuit of the causative agent of the disease generated keen competition in the Americas and Europe. The announcement in 1897 by Giuseppe Sanarelli, director of the Institute for Experimental Hygiene at the University of Montevideo, of his discovery of the causative agent of yellow fever, spurred an intense debate among the nascent American bacteriological community.[115]

Following the rules of etiological verification set out by Robert Koch and others, Sanarelli isolated the germ he had named *bacillus icteroides*, cultured it, and then injected the bacillus into laboratory animals. As a further test, he inoculated five patients from a quarantine station in Montevideo with an inactivated, filtered solution of the bacterium and then claimed to have produced in these patients the "imposing anatomical and symptomatological retinue" of typical yellow fever, including: "The fever, congestions, haemorrhages, vomiting, steatosis of the liver, cephalagia, rachialgia, nephritis, anuria, uraemia, icterus, delirium, collapse."[116] The fact that Sanarelli's claim to have discovered the causative agent of yellow fever was largely discredited by 1902 should not obscure the approbation with which his report was received within the American medical community and abroad. Walter Reed, whose own work on yellow fever in Havana had established the insect vector of the disease, wrote in 1902 of Sanarelli's discovery: "No more important achievement in scientific investigation has been claimed since Koch's announcement in 1882 of the discovery of the bacillus of tuberculosis."[117]

Discovery was not the critical issue for Leffingwell, however. Rather than the scientific import of the work, he seized upon the human dimensions of Sanarelli's inoculations and their implications for the doctor-patient relationship. "Whether men, women, or children, it was necessary that they should be ignorant, so that they should not be able to connect their future agonies with the kind old man who had simply pricked them with a needle; they must be so poor and friendless that no one would care to interest the authorities in their behalf; and they must be absolutely in the experimenter's power."[118] The willingness of physicians to use their patients in performing experiments, Leffingwell believed, signified a set of profoundly altered priorities. Where once traditions of medical paternalism and beneficence had held sway, commitment to science now took pride of place.

The American antivivisection movement developed in concert with several related and overlapping reforms in the second half of the nineteenth century, including the animal protection movement, the anticruelty to children movement, and the temperance crusade. Antivivisectionists perceived an intimate relationship between cruelty to animals and cruelty to human beings. Committed to protecting laboratory animals, they construed their responsibility broadly to include urban animals, food animals, wild animals used for clothing and decoration, and vulnerable human beings in medical research. Characterized by high levels of female involvement, the antivivisection movement attempted to reform humane education for children and the medical curriculum to include concern for the vulnerable.

Sanarelli's experiments with yellow fever quickened the humane movement's interest in the human subjects of medical research. Other experiments involving children and hospitalized patients soon joined Sanarelli's injections in antivivisectionist catalogues of human vivisections. Stories about physicians who experimented on children because they were "cheaper than animals" and reports of "murder in the name of science" in Baltimore and Boston led to bitter confrontations between the antivivisectionists and the leaders of the American medical profession.

Chapter Three

The American Medical Association
and the Defense of Research

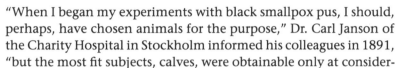 "When I began my experiments with black smallpox pus, I should, perhaps, have chosen animals for the purpose," Dr. Carl Janson of the Charity Hospital in Stockholm informed his colleagues in 1891, "but the most fit subjects, calves, were obtainable only at considerable cost."[1] The expense of acquiring and maintaining the calves led the Swedish physician to make his experiments instead upon fourteen children provided through the "kind permission" of the head physician of a nearby foundlings' home.[2] "Foundlings Cheaper than Animals" was the title of the Washington Humane Society's pamphlet introducing Janson's use of orphans to American readers.[3] Together with reports of other clinical investigations in which orphans, dying patients, and newly delivered mothers and infants received experimental injections, the Swedish vaccine trials became a prime exhibit in the antivivisection movement's indictment of "murder in the name of science."

The leaders of the organized medical profession were obliged to defend medical research when, from 1896 to 1900, charges that American physicians had experimented on vulnerable patients were thrust into the campaign to restrict animal experimentation at the federal level. There was much at stake. Leaders of the American Medical Association worried that such accusations would tarnish the new cultural authority of orthodox medicine.[4] Researchers feared that the loss of public support would create obstacles to experiments with both animals and humans. Believing that the abuse of patients in scientific research was rare and suspicious of antivivisectionist motives for highlighting human vivisection, defenders of research focused on exposing antivivisectionist errors, garblings, and deliberate misrepresentations in reports of human experimentation.

The medical profession's decision to deflect allegations of human vivisection and to dismiss legislative efforts to establish protections for human subjects was neither the result of ignorance nor the product of unfamiliarity with the ethical problems posed by the use of human beings in biomedical research. American physicians were aware of these issues; leaders of the medical profession were familiar with antivivisectionist critiques that emphasized the invasion of human rights that involuntary experimentation entailed. Leaders of the profession believed, however, that both patient interests and professional concerns would be best served by preserving free access to animals for medical research. In 1916 the leading defenders of research reconsidered this stance. In the wake of controversy over Hideyo Noguchi's clinical trials involving orphans and Udo Wile's "dental drill" experiments on insane patients, leaders of the American Medical Association considered adopting in its code of ethics an explicit provision about human experimentation.

In 1896 the American antivivisection movement began a campaign to restrict animal experimentation at the federal level. Passage of a bill that would ensure some protections for the animal subjects of experiments in the District of Columbia and the other research institutions of the federal government, antivivisectionists believed, would be useful in achieving similar laws at the state and local level.[5] Buoyed by the support of several influential legislators in the United States Congress, as well as the backing of the Woman's Christian Temperance Union, the antivivisection movement was confident about the future.

The Washington strategy accommodated both the reform and the abolitionist wings of the antivivisection movement. Like their English counterparts, who regarded the British Cruelty to Animals Act of 1876 as the first step toward the eventual elimination of all animal experiments, American abolitionists Mary Lovell and Caroline White explicitly countenanced the gradualist policy of regulation as a politically expedient "entering wedge" for abolition.[6] Vivisection reformers welcomed the opportunity to license researchers and to limit painful procedures on animals.

Jacob H. Gallinger (1837–1918), senior Republican senator from New Hampshire, was critical to the success of the antivivisection campaign. Although he had a reputation as a political conservative, Gallinger championed such reform causes as temperance and female suffrage. He was influential in the congressional passage of the Eighteenth Amendment (national prohibition) and the Nineteenth Amendment (women's suffrage).[7] Gallinger's colleagues respected his power as chair of the Committee on Pensions and they deferred to his medical expertise: after receiving medical degrees from the Cincinnati Medical Institute and the New York Homeopathic College, Gallinger had served as the surgeon general of New Hampshire, relinquishing the practice of medicine when he entered the House of Representatives in 1885.[8] In 1896, as chair of the Senate Committee on the District of Columbia, he presided at the public hearings on the cruelty to animals legislation.

The cruelty to animals bill, introduced by Senator James MacMillan of Michigan, closely followed the example of the successful British act of 1876. Even the name of the proposed legislation echoed the British model, although such critics as William Henry Welch claimed that American antivivisectionists had deliberately mislabeled the bill as cruelty to animals legislation when it was only intended to restrict animal experimentation.[9] The proposal set conditions for animal vivisectors similar to those required of British experimenters. The bill called for licensure of any person intending to experiment on animals and expressly proscribed the use of curare as an anesthetic. If granted by the Commissioners of the District of Columbia, the license would permit only those experiments deemed "useful for saving or prolonging life or alleviating suffering" and those intended to extend medical knowledge. Explicitly banned were vivisectional demonstrations for schoolchildren and the general public. Demonstrations for medical students required confirmation that the experiment would provide useful information for medical science. Additional certification, and evidence that no other animal could suffice, was necessary for permission to experiment on cats, dogs, horses, asses, and mules.[10]

After a session before the Civic Commissioners, the Senate Committee on the District of Columbia held public hearings on the revised proposal in 1896. Proponents of the bill marshaled impressive public support. In addition to animal welfare organizations and the WCTU, backers of the bill cited the patronage of six Supreme Court justices, a number of eminent Protestant and Catholic leaders, and such notable academics as John Bascom, emeritus president of the University of Wisconsin. A lengthy list of physicians—regulars, homeopaths, and eclectics—also endorsed passage of the bill.[11]

The widespread support for the bill disturbed medical educators and the leaders of the organized medical profession. On a practical level, maintaining unrestricted access to dogs, cats, horses, asses, rabbits, rats, and guinea pigs was of obvious importance to physiologists and pharmacologists, who required large numbers of animals for research. Any interference with the acquisition of animals was likely to cost additional time and money.[12] British physiologists, whose experiments on animals were regulated by the 1876 Cruelty to Animals Act, warned their American colleagues to anticipate difficulties and delays.[13]

Ambiguities in the proposal alarmed leaders of organized medicine. The legislation was vague in several crucial areas. The proposal did not specify, for example, the criteria for determining whether an experiment would lead to "useful knowledge" or even what "useful knowledge" might be. The bill as written also outlawed experiments on animals in order to acquire manual skill in performing surgical operations, as well as experiments to confirm the findings of other investigators.[14]

American researchers and their medical allies had more than a pragmatic investment in the protection of animal experimentation, however. The vivisection of animals had become a potent emblem of the reforms in medical therapeutics and medical education championed by the leaders of organized medicine and their allies in the laboratory. In the years between 1870 and 1910 the laboratory grew increasingly essential to the definition of medical education and the image of medical practice. Although the initial efforts to integrate laboratory science and methods into the medical curriculum in the 1870s were halting and their outcome uncertain, the trend toward laboratory scientific medicine in the 1890s was unmistakable.[15]

In the 1870s Charles W. Eliot's reforms at the Harvard Medical School, including the establishment of an assistant professorship in physiology and required laboratory training for medical students, rankled many of the clinical faculty.[16] The elevation of the laboratory sciences at the apparent expense of clinical instruction made the methodological tool of physiology—the vivisection of animals—a ready target for resistance to Eliot's reforms. One of the Harvard president's most vocal critics was the eminent Boston surgeon Henry Jacob Bigelow. Bigelow disputed the therapeutic optimism promoted by advocates of laboratory science and warned that reliance on the "chamber of torture and horrors" directly jeopardized the welfare of patients. "Watch the students at a vivisection," Bigelow soberly advised in an 1871 address on medical education: "It is the blood and suffering, not the science, that rivets their breathless attention. If hospital service makes young students less tender of suffering, vivisection deadens their humanity and begets indifference to it."[17] Although some American clinicians continued to harbor misgivings, an investment in laboratory science flourished among educational reformers, who pursued the rhetoric of research with remarkable intensity.[18]

By the 1890s, prominent medical educators shared a commitment to scientific medical education and laboratory instruction. The reforms in medical education undertaken at Harvard and other medical schools received dramatic reinforcement from the opening of the Johns Hopkins University School of Medicine in 1893.[19] Hopkins medical students not only met higher standards for admission, they also received extensive laboratory instruction in the basic sciences and clinical experience in the first American clerkships. In the course of preparing his infamous survey of medical education, Abraham Flexner measured all other medical schools against the Hopkins ideal and found them seriously deficient.[20]

Integrating the new disciplines of bacteriology and immunology into medical education and practice required large numbers of animal subjects.[21] The initial demonstrations of the new paradigm of the germ theory of disease involved animal diseases; the discovery and verification of the etiological agents of anthrax, a cattle disease, and chicken cholera, prepared the way for identification of the germs of human diseases. By the 1890s bacteriologists had identified the germs of tuberculosis, gonorrhea, leprosy, malaria, bubonic plague, typhoid, and diphtheria. These identifications in turn fostered the development of diagnostic tests, vaccines, and antitoxins for treatment of these diseases. Animals were necessary adjuncts in the development of these products, and in training medical students in their use.[22]

The animal body also became an important medium for pharmacology in the 1890s. Tests of both new and traditional drugs performed on animals generated a reliable and universalizable body of knowledge that provided one solution to the therapeutic disarray that had characterized American medicine in the mid-nineteenth century.[23] Transformed by John J. Abel, who joined the Hopkins faculty in 1893, pharmacology increasingly supplanted the more traditional *materia medica* in American medical schools. Rather than simply learning the names and sources of herbs, minerals, and other medicinal agents, Abel's medical students observed the action of drugs in living organisms. They learned to anesthetize dogs and rabbits and to perform surgical procedures on the animals.[24]

Any interference with the use of animals for research and teaching obviously threatened the therapeutic promises of scientific medicine and the professional aspirations of academic physicians and the clinical elite. Earlier efforts, in the 1880s and 1890s, to restrict animal experimentation had encouraged several medical societies to form committees to defend research interests. For the most part, these groups remained dormant until some impending legislation required committee members to contact law-makers or to appear at sessions of the legislature and speak against proposals to abolish or restrict animal experimentation. The New York State Medical Society organized the first explicit committee on experimental medicine, for example, in response to Henry Bergh's 1880 effort to abolish experimentation on live animals in New York.[25] Proposals to restrict animal experimentation in medical schools came before the Massachusetts legislature in the 1890s and prompted the Boston Society of Medical Sciences to form a defense committee. Chaired by Henry Bowditch, this group successfully defeated attempts to restrict animal experimentation in Massachusetts in 1896; and it was later joined by a statewide coalition of physicians, investigators, and educators committed to the protection of medical research.[26]

The 1896 decision by antivivisectionists to focus their efforts on the District of Columbia, as part of a national strategy to achieve restrictions on animal vivisection, caught the research community by surprise. Surgeon General George Sternberg hastily summoned investigators to appear at Senator Gallinger's initial hearing on MacMillan's cruelty to animals bill. The strong showing by the animal protection community inspired the research community to greater vigilance on the national front. Although the American Medical Association would in 1898 appoint a standing committee on national legislation in response to the vivisection issue, the threat in 1896 demanded immediate action.[27] William Henry Welch, dean of the Hopkins Medical School, and William Williams Keen, an eminent Philadelphia surgeon, quickly volunteered to repulse the antivivisectionist attack.

One of the strongest advocates of laboratory science in the United States, Welch guided organized medicine's response to the Washington proposals from 1896 to 1901.[28] Welch's training and education were exemplary of an emerging career pattern for medical scientists in the second half of the nineteenth century. After he received his medical degree from the College of Physicians and Surgeons in 1875, he devoted two years to postgraduate study in Germany and Austria. Upon return to the United States he endeavored to replicate his European experience, organizing, for example, the first American laboratory course in pathology. In 1884 he accepted Daniel Coit Gilman's invitation to participate in the new experiment in medical education at the Johns Hopkins University School of Medicine. At the medical school (which did not officially open until 1893), Welch introduced into American medicine the techniques of Robert Koch, the leading German bacteriologist. As part of Welch's efforts to foster the laboratory medical sciences in America, he founded in 1896 a journal for the publication of original American research. Although Welch feared that he would be unable to obtain manuscripts of sufficient quality for the journal, he was soon overwhelmed by papers of impressive quality being submitted to his *Journal of Experimental Medicine*.[29] Animal experimentation, Welch argued, was critical to the success of laboratory medicine; antivivisection jeopardized its bright future.

Welch observed with dismay the favorable reception of the 1896 proposal to restrict animal experimentation. He learned that such prominent supporters of the proposal as Supreme Court Justice David Brewer had lent their support in the belief that the act represented a compromise measure acceptable to the medical profession.[30] Fearing that others similarly assumed that the medical profession condoned the "cruelty-to-animals compromise," Welch entered the political arena. He instituted a letter-writing campaign involving respected physicians in every state, particularly the family doctors of individual senators, in order "to deluge the Senate with protests" against the MacMillan bill. He solicited the help of a number of scientific and medical organizations throughout the country and pursued personal channels of persuasion all the way to the White House, preparing himself, if necessary, to appeal to President Grover Cleveland for a veto.

The vote on the MacMillan bill was postponed because of the Spanish-American War, but in 1899 Gallinger supported a similar proposal, "Senate Bill 34: For the Further Prevention of Cruelty to Animals in the District of Columbia." On 21 February 1900, Gallinger and a subcommittee of the Senate Committee of the District of Columbia again heard testimony for and against animal experimentation, including repeated references to human experimentation. This time Welch and the defenders of research arranged an impressive showing of eminent medical authorities who were opposed to regulation of animal experimentation.[31]

Welch received considerable support from William Williams Keen, who was president of the American Medical Association in 1899–1900.[32] Keen traced his support for animal experimentation to his own surgical experiences in the preantiseptic era. After only one year at the Jefferson Medical College, Keen had practiced as a military surgeon during the first battle of Bull Run, in 1861, where the "dreadful" surgical conditions included wounds swarming with squirming maggots.[33] Impressed by the "surgical revolution" inaugurated by Joseph Lister's introduction of the principles of antisepsis in surgery, Keen considered the attempts to restrict animal experimentation as "a serious menace to progress, to life, and to health."[34] Informed by Lord Lister that had the restrictions of the 1876 British Cruelty to

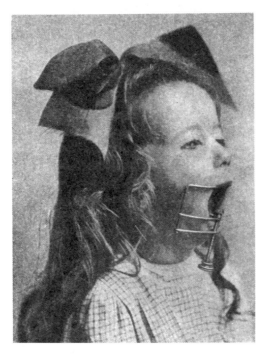

Surgeon William Williams Keen's granddaughter, wearing a mouth gag to illustrate that some medical procedures looked more painful than they were. From W. W. Keen, *Animal Experimentation and Medical Progress* (Boston, 1914).

Animals Act been in effect, they would have curtailed the animal experiments necessary to the discovery of antisepsis, Keen determined to oppose regulation of animal experimentation in the United States at all costs.[35]

Keen, Welch, and a parade of expert witnesses from Johns Hopkins, Harvard Medical School, and the United States government testified on behalf of animal experimenters. Welch even arranged for a testimonial from a respected female physician, Mary Putnam Jacobi, persuading her to appear as a representative of the "humane sex."[36] Opponents of Senate Bill 34 cited letters from such distinguished British investigators as Sir Michael Foster and Lord Joseph Lister, together with testimonials from medical and scientific societies. The committee's concerns about ambiguities in the proposal, along wiith Welch's politicking and the endorsements of medical and scientific societies, quashed the bill.[37]

The public support for proposals to regulate animal experimentation at first glance seems to contradict historical claims about the increasing cultural authority of science in general and of medical science in particular in late-nineteenth-century America.[38] It is tempting to dismiss such support as the result of prejudice and a lamentable ignorance about science, but the simple equation of antivivisection with anti-science flattens an understanding of the multiple, and in the late nineteenth century fluid, meanings of medical science. Antivivisectionists themselves at times embraced an idealized science, a search for truth, even as they rejected the privileging of the pursuit of knowledge over moral claims.[39]

The Supreme Court justices, clergymen, academics, and temperance activists who supported the regulation of animal experimentation did not categorically reject medical science nor did they brand all experimenters as cruel, sadistic brutes. They did favor a seemingly judicious approach to animal experimentation that allowed investigators to conduct research even as it afforded some protection for the animal subjects. The regulation of a practice as emotionally charged as animal vivisection appealed to these Americans in light of a characteristically Progressive optimism that the interests of all concerned could be best served by a supervisory bureaucracy.[40] The state, rather than an individual medical school or investigator, was considered the appropriate overseer of animal welfare. Many of the supporters of the MacMillan bill were no doubt surprised at being labeled unscientific, and they were unprepared for the vehement opposition of Welch, Keen, and their colleagues.

The medical support for the MacMillan bill and subsequent proposals reflected persistent misgivings on the part of a number of practicing physicians about the "undue importance" accorded new findings in bacteriology and the new emphasis on laboratory-based physiological instruction.[41] One conceptual objection to animal experimentation was based on species relationship. The widespread acceptance of Darwinian ideas about evolutionary descent encouraged a new sense of kinship between humans and other animals, yet the indisputable differences between human and nonhuman animals were pointed to by some physicians questioning the utility of a medical science grounded in mistaken correlations between animal function and human experience.[42] "No sufficient analogies exist in the animal kingdom from which to draw useful conclusions," argued one writer.[43] Experiments on guinea pigs and dogs would be essential to formulating treatments for those animals, such physicians conceded, but treating human patients necessitated clinical experience with human beings.[44] Although some of the intraprofessional resistance to analogical knowledge arose from a conflation of anatomical structure and physiological function, differing pharmacological responses among species raised problematic questions about the safety of minimizing species' variations.

Such objections aside, critics of laboratory science questioned whether anything of use for medical therapy had resulted from animal experimentation. The new science of bacteriology, heavily grounded in animal studies,

had contributed to understanding the etiology of such diseases as gonorrhea and plague, but prophylactic agents and therapies lagged persistently
behind the isolation of causative agents. Acknowledging that "physicians
too often get the impression that research is wholly and purely of theoretical value," one medical editor in 1903 emphasized the clinical value of
bacteriological examination of the blood, even as he promised that "from
the enormous mass of laboratory research there is sure to result sooner or
later knowledge that can be placed before the physician with the assurance
that it is a help in his efforts to recognize and cure disease."[45] Professional
misgivings about the germ theory of disease also reflected the lack of consensus about standards of etiological proof and irreproducible discoveries of
disease germs. When Fritz Schaudinn and Erich Hoffman reported their
discovery of the spirochete of syphilis in 1905, medical editors praised the
Germans for the modesty of their announcement, a trait they had found
lacking in the more than twenty previous claimants to the discovery of the
etiological agent of syphilis.[46] The "disastrous experience" of Robert Koch's
prematurely heralded cure for tuberculosis in 1891 prompted some American physicians to receive the discovery of diphtheria antitoxin in 1894 with
skepticism, if not outright hostility.[47]

The defenders of medical research insisted that the physicians who
supported proposals to regulate animal experimentation were largely older
practitioners, small town doctors, and various irregulars.[48] Even if being
from a small town equaled small-mindedness, their marginal status may
not have prevented these physicians from accurately reading cultural attitudes toward animal experimentation, however. The twentieth-century
edition of D. W. Cathell's popular guide to medical practice, for example,
advised readers that animal experimentation was permissible as a means of
benefiting human beings and advancing medical science. Nonetheless, "the
useless and unjustifiable repetition of physiological and pathological experiments, made merely to gratify curiosity or to illustrate known facts, that
require vivisection of animals," the guide warned, "is, by many, considered
cruel and will not add much to your reputation."[49] Proposals that limited
experimenters to projects that involved new experiments only (rather than
the repetition of experiments whose outcome was already known) appealed
to some physicians because they promoted mutually beneficial ends: they
allowed medical science to advance; they prohibited useless animal suffering; and they pacified parties concerned about animal welfare in medical
laboratories.

Closely linked to the discussion of animal experimentation was the issue of human vivisection. At the Senate committee hearings in 1900, Senator Gallinger repeatedly questioned medical witnesses about the relationship between human and animal experimentation and demanded that the American Medical Association respond to the exploitation of vulnerable human beings by vivisecting doctors.

The plans to thrust human vivisection into the animal experimentation hearings were laid in advance. Senator Gallinger entered into the minutes of the Senate a document describing several cases of nontherapeutic human experimentation. Senate Document 78 (as it became known) included accounts of Sanarelli's yellow fever experiments, as well as extracts from the published papers of three American physicians.[50] In order to understand the vehemence of the human vivisection controversy, some familiarity with these cases is required.

The earliest example of human vivisection cited in Senate Document 78 involved experiments with syphilis in the Hawaiian Islands. In 1883 George L. Fitch, an American physician serving as resident physician to the leper settlement on Molokai Island, conducted experiments intended to demonstrate that leprosy and syphilis were actually manifestations of the same disease. To substantiate his claims, he inoculated six young girls suffering from leprosy with the "virus of syphilis."[51] The failure of the children to develop syphilitic symptoms lent credence, Fitch claimed, to his theory of the essential unity of syphilis and leprosy. Fitch repeated his experiments on more than a dozen men and women from the leper settlement and published his findings in an American medical journal after his return to the mainland.[52]

Less exotic than experiments with Hawaiian lepers were trials with thyroid extract on patients in a Baltimore mental hospital. In 1897 Henry J. Berkley, an associate in neuropathology at the Johns Hopkins University, in order to determine the toxicity of one of the best-known commercial preparations of thyroid extract, selected for study eight patients who "with one exception had either passed or were about to pass the limit of time in which recovery could be confidently expected."[53] He administered the extract in gradually increasing doses that invariably produced weight loss and disturbances of the circulation. Some patients experienced digestive upsets, irritability, and great mental excitement. According to Berkley, one woman, Olivia P., age 27, lost weight very rapidly and on the twelfth day, passed into "a state of frenzy."[54] Although her thyroid regimen was discontinued, Olivia P.'s symptoms of mental and motor distress persisted. Despite the application of baths, narcotics, and systematic exercise, her excitement continued until her death seven weeks later. The cause of death was listed as acute miliary tuberculosis, an assessment based on clinical evidence alone, since no autopsy was permitted.[55] Berkley concluded from his trials with thyroid extract that the administration of even the purest of the commercially available thyroid tablets had the potential to harm the health and life of the patient.[56]

The third American case in Senate Document 78 involved "the vivisection of children in Boston." In August 1896 Arthur H. Wentworth, assistant in diseases of children at Harvard Medical School and out-patient physician to the Children's Hospital, reported the results of experimental tapping of the subarachnoid space of the spinal cords of sick infants and children.[57] Although lumbar puncture had been introduced in 1891 as a therapeutic procedure for relief in cases of hydrocephalus, Wentworth's punctures were admittedly experimental in nature. Convinced of the diagnostic value of examination of the fluid obtained by spinal puncture, Wentworth began conducting experiments to determine whether a disturbance in the normal pressure of the spinal fluid was dangerous to a child. He attempted "control experiments on normal cases," explaining: "The diagnostic value of puncture of the subarachnoid space is so evident that I considered myself justified in incurring some risk in order to settle the question of its danger. If it proved to be harmless, then one need not wait until a patient became moribund before resorting to it."[58] Wentworth subsequently performed more than forty-five punctures on children whose ages ranged from a few hours to several years. The punctures, some performed shortly before or at the time of death, did not harm the children in Wentworth's opinion, although the "momentary pain of the puncture" did cause some children to shrink back and to cry aloud.[59]

The human vivisections cited in the Senate document reappeared in a pamphlet issued by the American Humane Association.[60] Augmented by newspaper accounts of European experiments involving the grafting of cancerous material onto anesthetized female patients; of inoculations of human beings with solutions of syphilitic organisms, filtered peritoneal pus, and tuberculin; and of Janson's inoculation trials of "black smallpox pus" on foundlings, the pamphlet elicited surprise and intense scrutiny at the Senate hearing on the proposed cruelty to animals bill in 1900.[61] At that hearing, Senator Gallinger, in his capacity as chairman, raised the issue of human experimentation with several of the eminent medical witnesses who were appearing against the bill. He questioned the doctors about Berkley's experiments with thyroid extract, which had been reported in the

Bulletin of the Johns Hopkins Hospital.[62] Although the distinguished Johns Hopkins clinician William Osler denied that Berkley's trials had any connection with Hopkins Hospital (the tests had been conducted in the Bay View Insane Asylum in Baltimore), he condemned improper experimentation on patients.[63] Osler insisted that the medical profession absolutely opposed nontherapeutic experiments upon patients, and he challenged the humane movement's assertion that physicians condoned such immoral practices. On the subject of Sanarelli's yellow fever experiments he quoted a professor from a leading medical college who in 1898 had strongly censured the Italian bacteriologist:

> The work of Sanarelli has been marred by a series of unjustifiable experiments upon men which should receive the unqualified condemnation of the profession. The limitations of deliberate experimentation upon human beings should be clearly defined. Voluntarily, if with full knowledge, a fellow-creature may submit to certain tests, just as a physician may experiment upon himself. Drugs, the value of which has been carefully tested in animals and are found harmless may be tried on patients, since in this way alone may progress be made, but deliberate experiments such as Sanarelli carried on with cultures of known and tested virulence, and which were followed by nearly fatal illnesses, are simply criminal.[64]

Though he had in fact written the condemnation himself, Osler refused to name the author for Gallinger. The statement had appeared as a footnote to the discussion of yellow fever in Osler's text, *The Principles and Practice of Medicine.*[65]

Although some antivivisectionists continued to dispute Osler's implicit claim that only marginal physicians experimented on patients, his impassioned testimony at the Senate hearings may have appeased critics who complained that the medical profession failed to criticize human vivisectors.[66] William Williams Keen's testimony, however, provoked intense controversy. In one of his thirty-seven interruptions of Keen's testimony to the committee, Gallinger asked the surgeon about vivisectors who "progress[ed] from the brute creation to the human creation" in making human experiments.[67] Although Keen informed the senator that the humane association's pamphlet included a number of experiments that he would absolutely condemn, he insisted that only two of the alleged experiments occurred in America. (Keen did not include Fitch's syphilis inoculations because their occurrence antedated the American annexation of Hawaii in 1898.) Rather than dwell on the experiments he regarded as unethical, Keen sharply criticized the humane society for a series of vague references and garbled, inaccurate accounts.

Keen's Senate testimony prompted a series of rancorous exchanges between Keen and the president of the American Humane Association, James M. Brown, in the pages of antivivisectionist magazines and medical journals. Whereas the antivivisectionists demanded recognition of research abuse of patients by experimenting doctors, the leaders of the organized medical profession intently pursued freedom from restrictions on animal experimentation. Hostile exchanges, extravagant accusations, and vehement denials eclipsed any candid public discussion of the moral problems posed by clinical and laboratory research.[68]

For William Keen and the medical defenders of unrestricted animal experimentation, the critical task in the human vivisection controversy was to discredit antivivisectionist claims that physicians had performed dangerous experiments on unsuspecting patients. Keen, Welch, and their colleagues devoted considerable energy to developing the most effective responses to the charges of human vivisection. Their rhetorical strategies consistently focused on antivivisectionist errors and exaggerations. In his exchange with James Brown, Keen emphasized antivivisectionist shortcomings rather than his professional concerns about experimenting doctors.

Almost from the start, the defenders of research were predisposed to dismiss accusations of human vivisection as unfounded and exaggerated. The unbridled antagonism and unbalanced characterization that marked much of the antivivisectionist literature encouraged their hostility. Antivivisectionist tracts frequently described research laboratories as "scientific hells," "torture houses," "halls of agony," and "temples of torment." References to medical investigators as "devils incarnate," "human monsters," "criminals," and "arch-fiends" hardly facilitated an unprejudiced hearing by medical researchers on the accusations of immoral human experimentation.[69]

The antivivisectionist style of debate also encouraged defenders of research to dismiss accusations of human vivisection. Antivivisectionist compilers relied on illustrative sentences or paragraphs taken directly from scientific publications. They selectively edited passages, and added graphic titles, thereby prompting defenders of medical research to cry foul. Complained one professor of biology, "[Antivivisectionists] simply select those sentences which, to a diseased imagination, savor of the sensational, deliberately omitting the setting of the sentences quoted, and then publish these statements with innumerable additions, exaggerations, and material of their own manufacture."[70] Although the compiler of the human vivisection pamphlet and the president of the American Humane Association both prefaced their remarks by explaining that limitations of space made it impossible to print the full details of the human experiments, Keen attacked their "literary forgeries" of medical texts, committed in the attempt to substantiate the reality of human vivisection.[71]

Typical of antivivisectionist misrepresentation, in Keen's estimation, was the humane society's use of the title "Senate Document" in the preface to the abstracts of human vivisection: "A document recently issued by the United States Government (Senate Document, No. 78) contains matter of such great importance that it has been decided to reprint that portion which treats of HUMAN VIVISECTION, and to place a copy in the hand of those who contribute to the formation and guidance of public opinion in the United States."[72] Keen complained to William Welch that uninformed readers would infer from this statement that the report on human vivisection appeared with the sanction of the federal government, when in fact it was merely part of a group of documents offered as testimony into the records of the Senate. Welch advised the surgeon that just because some "guileless persons" might be deceived, he could not support a charge of deception on the part of the secretary or president of the humane society.[73] Undeterred, Keen criticized the humane society for using the phrase "Senate Document," a usage that he considered to be illustrative of the misrepresentations and inaccuracies he found characteristic of antivivisectionist literature. That Keen and Welch did not always agree on the best strategy to frustrate their critics is evident from their exchanges. More compelling than their occasional disagreement, however, was their willingness to mull over even minor word changes to thwart their common enemy.

Keen's animus toward the humane society may have been due in part to his knowledge of the compiler of Senate Document 78, "A. Tracy." In 1901 Francis Stuart, a Brooklyn physician, informed Keen that A. Tracy was the pen name of the well-known vivisection reformer Albert Tracy Leffingwell, an old adversary.[74] Leffingwell's decision to use a pen name angered Keen, who suspected that Leffingwell had written the strongly worded review of Keen's responses to James Brown contained in the report.[75] Although he subsequently discovered that not Leffingwell but a former president of the Brooklyn Polytechnic (where Leffingwell had once taught physiology using vivisectional techniques) had written the review, Keen remained antagonistic to Leffingwell.[76]

Keen attacked the humane society for "either gross ignorance or wilful disregard of the truth" in making textual additions to accounts of human vivisection. The most outrageous instance of mistranslation, in William Keen's opinion, was the description of Schreiber's observations and experiments with tuberculin.[77] In the humane society pamphlet, a purportedly exact translation of the medical report of Schreiber's tuberculin injections began with the German physician's startling statement that it was difficult to obtain healthy children for experiments; the account further suggested that Schreiber deliberately infected the children with tuberculosis.[78] Keen pointedly observed that these sentences did not appear in the original text but were "additions made out of the whole cloth." Moreover, he argued, the pamphlet misconstrued the purpose and safety of Schreiber's research. The injections were intended for the diagnosis of tuberculosis, a necessary first step in treating consumptive children.[79]

Keen criticized the humane society for omissions from, as well as additions to, their "representative" medical texts. He objected strongly to the manner in which the experiments of two American physicians were presented. Deliberate omissions in the pamphlet's version, Keen insisted, fostered the false impression that both Wentworth's pediatric patients and the inmates of the Baltimore asylum where Berkley conducted trials of thyroid extract had died as a result of their research participation. Although he privately informed Gallinger that he thoroughly disapproved of Wentworth's punctures, Keen publicly focused on the "deliberate distortions" in the presentation of the results of Wentworth's lumbar punctures. For example, in one case a female infant aged four months received a spinal puncture on 17 January 1896 and died four days later.[80] The pamphlet deleted Wentworth's note that no symptoms attended the operation and that the infant had died "from the widespread changes common to infantile wasting." For several other infants who died after lumbar puncture, the medical cause of death was also missing from the pamphlet. "The inference from the pamphlet's 'brief abstracts' of these cases is clearly, and it seems to me by these omissions was meant to be, that the deaths were due to the lumbar punctures," Keen observed caustically, "whereas the evidence is that the deaths were due to other causes, and in two instances the operation is expressly stated not to have done any harm."[81]

Similar omissions of relevant information marked the discussion of Berkley's trials of thyroid extract. Berkley named the cause of death for two patients who died after administration of the thyroid extract, and Keen complained that this information did not appear in the human vivisection pamphlets. Neglecting to include the cause of death (as in the case of Olivia P.), Keen argued, led readers to infer that the patients had died as a result of the thyroid tablets: "To say that this patient, who actually died of galloping consumption, died from the effects of the thyroid extract, which had not been given for seven weeks before death is as absurd as it would be to say she had died from the effects of moderate doses of laudanum given seven weeks before."[82] Even more damaging in Keen's eyes, however, was the conclusion appearing in Senate Document 78 that a female patient who had succumbed to acute miliary tuberculosis after receiving thyroid extract had been "scientifically murdered." The fact that this "piece of absurdity" was deleted from the subsequent humane society pamphlet Keen chose to interpret not as an attempt at accuracy on the part of the American Humane Association but as evidence of the inability of laypersons to interpret medical writings.[83]

Keen's public defense of the Baltimore physician's research did not reveal the considerable deliberation about the clinical trials of thyroid extract that had preceded it. References to "poisoning patients" and other careless language in Berkley's article, William Henry Welch frankly informed Keen, had created many difficulties: "The article, including its title, contains many most unfortunate phrases, and it never should have been published in the form in which it appeared."[84] Concern about adverse publicity from the thyroid extract trials prompted Welch to prepare a statement regarding Berkley's alleged human vivisections and to have it approved by the Medical Board of the Johns Hopkins Hospital.[85]

Most problematic in Welch's view was Berkley's reference to the administration of thyroid tablets as experiments rather than as medical therapy. The use of thyroid tablets at the Bay View Insane Asylum was not research, Welch argued, but an accepted treatment for mental disease for which there was ample justification. Welch noted that every application of a drug could be considered an experiment, but that Berkley had employed the usual therapeutic dosages of an accepted medication in order to benefit individual patients. Based on his experiments at the asylum, Berkley concluded that instead of being beneficial, the treatment might be injurious to some insane patients. Despite Berkley's findings, many physicians continued to recommend thyroid extract for the treatment of insanity.[86] "Berkley's mistake is in describing his tests of the treatment as 'experiments' and in talking about his patients being poisoned by the drug, etc.," Welch informed Keen, when in fact "he did nothing which others had not done before and are not doing now with apparently beneficial results."[87]

Stung by the criticism of an English physician who accused him of conducting "experiments on lunatics," Berkley had in 1897 offered a similar justification for his clinical trials with thyroid extract, in the *British Medical Journal*.[88] Berkley explained that rather than testing the gland extract on "incurable" patients, he had administered thyroid tablets to the eight patients in order "to give them a chance to recover their mental vigor, as they had either passed, or were about to pass the limit of time in which recovery could be confidently expected." Although he conceded that the wording of his original article was "in some ways unfortunate," he insisted that the trials were therapeutic attempts, not experimental investigations.[89]

For Berkley, Welch, and Keen, the clinical investigation of thyroid treatment was legitimate therapeutic research. No similar justification could be made for injecting the filtrate of the bacillus of yellow fever into hospital patients. Sanarelli performed the injections to verify the status of the microbe, not to benefit the patients. The discussion of Sanarelli's experiments in the Brown-Keen exchanges epitomized the frustrations both sides experienced in the debate. Brown and his compatriots sought the condemnation of the experiments by the medical profession. Even though Keen and Welch disapproved of Sanarelli's experiments on patients, their primary concern was maintaining a united front against the animal protectionists. Unlike William Osler who had openly denounced the Italian physician's research, Keen declined to criticize the experimenter publicly, reserving his criticism for antivivisectionists who misrepresented Sanarelli's research.

Keen's chief target in deflecting accusations of human vivisection against Sanarelli was again the inaccuracy with which the yellow fever serum experiments were reported. The compilers of the human vivisection pamphlet, who had relied on abstracts of Sanarelli's paper published in English and American journals, intimated that the experimental subjects had died as a result of their participation. William Welch sent Keen the citation and an abstract from the original Italian communication. Like Osler, Welch considered Sanarelli's experiments inexcusable, but the misrepresentation of the yellow fever research disturbed him. "I disapprove of Sanarelli's experiments on human beings," he privately informed Keen, "but the statement that he inoculated the germs of yellow fever or living bacteria of any kind and that any of these experiments ended fatally are false."[90]

The Italian account reported that none of the five patients injected with the filtrate had died as a result of the experiment. The two patients who received subcutaneous injections developed mild swellings, vomiting, and loss of appetite. Of the three patients receiving intravenous injections, two developed more significant symptoms and the fifth proved not susceptible to the infection.[91] Sanarelli had not, contrary to claims by antivivisection-ists, injected the actual germ of yellow fever, but a solution of the inacti-vated microbe. Welch did not address the fact that Sanarelli claimed to have produced yellow fever from these injections in his subjects. Given the anti-vivisectionists' inference that Sanarelli had "scientifically murdered" his patients, Welch was unsympathetic to the possibility that antivivisection-ists might understandably have confused the nature of the injections in light of Sanarelli's assertions about his experiments. In fact, Welch did not believe that Sanarelli had produced yellow fever. Like other members of the growing community of American bacteriologists, Welch believed that San-arelli had not isolated the causative bacillus of yellow fever, but some other pathogen. The relegation of Sanarelli's germ to a "bacteriological limbo" served in part to mitigate the experimenter's conduct.[92]

Using the absence of injury from participation in nontherapeutic re-search to excuse an investigator's use of human beings recurred in organized medicine's response to charges of human vivisection. It enabled defenders of research to avoid the messy issue of obtaining patient consent, and it diminished the potentially damaging allegation that physicians were sub-jecting unknowing participants to potential harms for scientific rather than therapeutic purposes. In his dispute with the American Humane Associa-tion, Keen maintained that patients had not been harmed by experimen-ters. He contended, for example, that none of the young girls whom Fitch had inoculated with syphilis had developed the disease. He did not mention that their participation might have entailed considerable risks for them.

Keen offered a similar explanation in the case of Karl Menge, a German investigator who reportedly injected into newborn infants pus from the abdominal cavity of a person who had died from peritonitis. Keen explained that after the sterilizing process, Menge's inoculations would "almost cer-tainly" have been harmless. The infants, at the university women's clinic in Leipzig, apparently suffered no ill effects as a result of the injections of staphylococci.[93] Voicing sentiments calculated to anger his opponents, Keen observed, "I have only words of condemnation for Menge's experi-ments, but to misrepresent them is scarcely less culpable than to perform them."[94] The absence of injury to the infants and the indictment of anti-vivisectionist misrepresentation took much of the sting out of Keen's criti-cism of the German physician's injections. William Welch took a similar stance in his comments on Carl Janson's experimenting on foundlings be-cause they were "cheaper than animals." Welch privately told Keen that such language, taken from an essentially accurate translation of Janson's remarks in the antivivisectionist pamphlet, cast the medical profession in a negative light and sounded "abominable." He maintained, nonetheless, that the Swedish physician's injections of sterilized vaccine lymph and sterilized blood serum (not smallpox virus) into children were "harmless enough."[95]

Wentworth's studies of lumbar puncture were also defended as harmless to the children who had undergone the experimental spinal taps. In Boston a unified defense of Wentworth's clinical trials became necessary when in 1900 they prompted the New England Anti-Vivisection Society to organize a statewide drive for restrictions on animal experimentation in Massachusetts. An extremely negative medical review of Wentworth's experiments that criticized the pediatrician for his "cruelty to the helpless" also worried the Boston-area defenders of animal research.[96] Henry Bowditch, Theobald Smith, and others active in the research committee of the Boston Society of Medical Sciences concluded that despite their clinical utility, Wentworth's trials would be difficult to justify. Although Wentworth had been scheduled to testify at the hearing on animal experimentation, he did not appear. After the hearing, he resigned his position at Harvard amid speculation that the university administration feared the accusations of human vivisection would hurt fund-raising efforts. Although Wentworth retained his position at the Children's Hospital, he believed that the incident damaged his academic career.[97]

In 1901 the American Humane Association issued an anonymous review of the "reality of human vivisection." Conceding that the original pamphlet had contained errors in transcription and translation from the original sources, the association nonetheless insisted that the suggestion that "non-injury to the victims" did not constitute "a substantial excuse for the deeds" and in no way mitigated either "the essential wickedness of the experiment, or the criminality of that physician or surgeon who can stoop to the commission of such infamous acts."[98] The physician's crime, claimed the humane society, was the instrumental use of an unsuspecting person for research purposes. The potential for risk and the actual harm patients suffered intensified the moral violation. Although the patients of Menge, Janson, and Fitch apparently suffered no ill effects, the word of an experimenting doctor could hardly be trusted as evidence of the lack of injury. Just as Keen challenged the veracity of any antivivisectionist account of human vivisection, this anonymous writer refused to accept the word of a physician that no harm to a research subject resulted from such experimental procedures. Suspicion and hostility were operating on both sides.[99]

Medical attempts to downplay the use of human beings in experiments
for the purposes of science, especially those involving the new sciences of
bacteriology and immunology, inflamed the AHA. The "disregard for human rights" that characterized both the experiments and William Keen's
attempts to minimize the violation of individuals offended them. Even
more disturbing to them was the researchers' apparent lack of sympathy for
the experimental subjects.

Keen criticized the omission from this new publicaiton of the fact that
Sanarelli had employed sterilized germ-free cultures of his bacillus; the AHA
countered by asking if the president of the American Medical Association
could not spare a few words of sympathy for the victims of Sanarelli's research. Keen had sarcastically referred to scientific assassinations in which
the subjects were so disobliging as to remain alive, and this struck the AHA
as inappropriate and unfeeling levity:

> If a child of Dr. Keen were thus unconsciously inoculated with "the carefully-
> filtered and sterilized *germ-free*" toxin of yellow fever and made to suffer day
> after day all the torments that Sanarelli has so vividly described; and if, after the
> fever had abated, a few "explorative punctures" were made in his liver and
> kidneys, ("*varie puncture esplorative dal fegato e dai reni*") revealing a profound
> fatty degeneration of the one and granular degeneration of the other, we are
> inclined to think that such endowment of his offspring with the beginnings of
> organic disease and the probabilities of shortened life would be regarded as
> "scientific assassination" even by the man who now scoffs at the phrase.[100]

The apparent lack of sympathy for experimental subjects and the clinical detachment with which physicians described experiments on human
beings was a recurrent theme in discussions of human vivisection. "Note
the cool, precise, heartless language in which experiments on helpless, de-
mented wards of the public are described," wrote one commentator on
Berkley's thyroid extract experiments. "Not the slightest hint that Dr.
Berkley—a teacher of men—was solicitous for the welfare of these insane
patients. . . . Simply a placing of science above morality in the hope that the
experimenter might feel the swelling of pride as he realized that he had
added another mite of knowledge to scientific research."[101] The ambition of
medical scientists and their evident insensitivity to human suffering made
securing legal protection for human subjects a goal of antivivisectionists.

In addition to the cruelty to animals bill, Senator Gallinger introduced
in 1900 a proposal for the regulation of human experimentation in the
District of Columbia. Senate Bill 3424 required the prior disclosure of an

investigator's purpose and procedures in any *nontherapeutic* experiment on human beings, as well as the written consent of the subjects. The bill expressly outlawed scientific experimentation on persons considered incapable of giving consent, including newborns and children under the age of twenty, pregnant women or women who had given birth in the previous year, the aged, the insane, the feeble-minded, and people with epilepsy.[102]

Medical critics rejected Gallinger's proposal as gratuitous and ignored the ethical compromise it implied. One medical commentator, especially insulted that the bill allowed "any experiments whatsoever made by medical students, physicians, surgeons, physiologists, or pathologists upon one another," suggested that the proposal was more in the nature of a practical joke than a matter of concern for the United States Senate.[103]

But the proposal to regulate human experimentation prompted a private appeal to Gallinger from William Keen, then president of the AMA. Keen characterized the two instances of human vivisection in America (Wentworth's lumbar punctures and Berkley's thyroid trials) as "entirely unjustifiable experimentation," even as he warned that such regulation of human experimentation would impose considerable hardship on the physicians in the District of Columbia. "You know how unreasonable patients are, especially if the result is not all that they anticipated," Keen reminded the Senator. "If the Bill 3424 becomes a law, it will inevitably give rise to a large number of suits on the ground of experiment." Given the rarity of human vivisection, Keen declared that physicians did not need an act of Congress. "The moral sense of the profession may well be relied upon to prevent any extension of such an objectionable method without any law to restrain it."[104]

Like William Henry Welch, William Williams Keen subordinated his personal disapproval of human vivisection to his public defense of medical experimentation. Buoyed by confidence in the ethical judgment of the medical profession and faith in animal experimentation as the means to medical progress, the proponents of research and their allies defended experimentation in medicine against accusations of abuse and cruelty. However, continuing accusations of human vivisection and fear that clinical researchers were, in fact, compromising patient welfare in the name of medical science led Keen and his colleagues to consider developing explicit rules for research involving human beings.

Chapter Four

Rules for Research:
Human Experimentation and the
AMA Code of Ethics

 In 1909 Walter Bradford Cannon, chair of the American Medical Association's Council on the Defense of Medical Research, circulated a set of rules among all American laboratories and medical schools that had reported using animals in research. The committee did not expect that the regulations would alter the care animals already received in the best institutions. The rules did "indicate, however, to newcomers in the laboratories, and to interested and intelligent people, the intent of the investigators and the precautions which they take against suffering."[1]

Forging consensus among investigators about a uniform code of regulations for animal experimentation was not without difficulty. After personally contacting the deans of seventy-nine medical schools, Cannon enthusiastically reported in March 1910 that thirty-seven schools and research institutes had agreed to adopt and enforce the rules and an additional twenty-two institutions had expressed willingness to implement the code. In a letter to Thomas Hughes, governor of New York, where an antivivisection proposal was pending in the state legislature, Cannon confidently predicted that before the year ended, the regulations would "probably be enforced in all the medical laboratories in the United States."[2]

Six years later, in 1916, Cannon proposed that similar guidelines be developed for clinical investigators and their human subjects. New charges of human vivisection from antivivisectionists and concern that young investigators were not respecting the rights of patients prompted Cannon's recommendation that the AMA amend its code of ethics to include the responsibilities of experimenters to patients. But the leaders of the organized medical profession and the research community could not agree.

Clinical investigators would continue to work without any formal guide-lines until the 1940s, when the AMA amended the code to require voluntary consent of the subject and prior animal testing.[3]

The decision to forgo requiring the patient's consent to experimenta-tion reflected some of the ambiguities in medical research on human beings in the early twentieth century. Distinguishing between therapeutic and nontherapeutic experiments, for example, was not always easy. Although deliberately exposing volunteers to mosquitoes infected with yellow fever was clearly nontherapeutic research, the use of control subjects in the devel-opment of new vaccines or diagnostic tests, a major focus of research in this period, presented greater difficulties for physicians. They also had questions about the details of patient consent: When a pediatrician conducted tests of a new vaccine in a state-sponsored orphanage was permission needed? Who should authorize the children's participation? Was patient permission real-ly necessary for such relatively benign procedures as urine testing or obtain-ing a small blood sample? Given the inequality of the doctor-patient rela-tionship and the patient's dependency, some physicians challenged the value of a patient's formal permission for experimentation. Providing the necessary information to enable the patient to make an informed decision, these investigators argued, would not only burden patients and their doc-tors but interfere with the vital progress of medical knowledge.

Pressure from antivivisectionists and continuing accusations of scien-tific exploitation encouraged Cannon to confront the issue of human ex-perimentation, but they did not foster a climate conducive to open discus-sions between the medical profession and the public. The defeat of the Washington campaigns to regulate both human and animal experimenta-tion had redoubled the antivivisectionists' focus on the "inevitable tenden-cy of vivisection" to result in human vivisection. But writing explicit rules for human experimentation promised to create more dilemmas than it might resolve.

Cannon's recommendation that rules for human research be circulated among the growing number of clinical investigators followed more than a decade of continuing accusations of human vivisection. Antivivisectionists sponsored a number of unsuccessful legislative proposals to regulate human experimentation. In 1902 Senator Gallinger reintroduced his measure to regulate human experimentation in the District of Columbia. The Mary-land state legislature briefly considered a similar bill during the same year. In 1905 and again in 1907 the Vivisection Reform Society, a Chicago-based group whose members included Senator Gallinger, James Cardinal Gibbons of Baltimore, Harvard philosopher William James, and Albert Leffingwell, urged passage of a bill in the Illinois state legislature "to prohibit such terrible experiments on children, insane persons and certain women as have been performed of late years" and to insure "that no experiment should be performed on any other human being without his intelligent written consent."[4] Sydney R. Taber, a Chicago attorney and secretary of the society, conceded that his organization did not anticipate success with the proposal but hoped to enlighten the public on the "dark subject" of human and animal vivisection.[5]

Reports in the medical literature and the popular press convinced Taber that earlier commentators had underestimated the extent of human vivisection. In 1906 he compiled a new catalog of human vivisections, including older reports by two physicians whose testimony had helped to defeat the Washington restrictions on animal experimentation. Taber labeled the "distinguished lady-physician" Mary Putnam Jacobi and Philadelphia surgeon William Williams Keen human vivisectors. Putnam Jacobi's demonstration of the effect of the drug atropine on a "rather robust woman in good health" for the students at the Woman's College of the New York Infirmary in 1873 helped earn her inclusion in Taber's list. He also condemned her research involving a "very healthy Irish boy, age 10." Although he conceded that Josie Nolan had escaped serious harm from Putnam Jacobi's study of the conditions affecting intracranial pressure in the boy's fractured skull, Taber criticized the instrumental use of children in research that promised no benefit for them.[6]

William Keen was also targeted as an example of the overzealous pursuit of medical science. In 1865 Keen, Silas Weir Mitchell, and George Morehouse had reported the results of a study of the effect of atropine and morphine on soldiers at an army hospital. Although Taber approved the experimental application of the drugs for the purpose of relieving the men's painful neuralgia, he criticized the experiments conducted on soldiers "free of fever" and on "men in very fair health, suspected of malingering."[7] Although the physicians insisted that the experiments were therapeutic in intent, and emphasized the absence of injury for the patients, Taber raised the issue of individual rights: "what moral right had these medical gentlemen thus to experiment upon the eye, the pulse, the brain of a single soldier of this Republic" without the subjects' knowledge?[8]

Taber raised a similar issue about the authority to conduct experiments on a prison population in the American-occupied Philippines. In 1906 Richard Pearson Strong, director of the Biological Laboratory of the Philippine

Bureau of Science, inoculated thirty-four inmates at Manila's Bilibid Prison with a contaminated cholera vaccine.[9] The vaccine-related deaths of thirteen prisoners prompted Senator Jacob Gallinger to request an official investigation to determine "whether any of the persons so experimented upon were previously informed of the dangerous and possibly fatal character of the experiments."[10] Although Secretary of War William Howard Taft confirmed that none of the prisoners was vaccinated against his will, Sydney Taber asked, "How many of the two thousand prisoners were informed at the time of the operation that it was their privilege to refuse inoculation without incurring punishment?"[11] The "sort of consent" obtained from the Filipino prisoners, Taber maintained, was similar to the permission granted by two "negro prisoners" in a New Orleans jail, who "consented" to a steady diet of molasses for five weeks (in order to determine whether the additive sulfuric acid was injurious). The prisoners reportedly did not "object to submitting themselves to the test, because it would not do any good if they did."[12]

In addition to experiments on soldiers and prisoners, Taber criticized the use of children in research conducted by a New Jersey physician, Joseph W. Stickler. Believing that just as inoculations of cowpox immunized human beings against smallpox, Stickler hoped that the inoculation of foot-and-mouth-disease would protect children from scarlet fever, a dreaded childhood disease. In 1887 he approached several physicians with his discovery, asking their permission to try his vaccine on their patients. After receiving rejections from the distinguished pediatrician Abraham Jacobi and several other doctors, Stickler injected himself and two young children with his vaccine. The protection of the inoculation was challenged by exposing the children to scarlet fever patients and their infected bed linens. The children did not develop scarlet fever, and descriptions of Stickler's experiments appeared in several American medical journals.[13]

If Stickler had confined the experiments to his own body, he would have earned the approval of most antivivisectionists. Investigators who studied themselves or adult volunteers generally received good reviews in the antivivisectionist press. In 1906 the *Journal of Zoophily* praised the publication of Russell Chittenden's "altogether honorable and useful work of scientific research" into the minimal daily protein requirements for healthy human beings. The director of the Sheffield Scientific School at Yale University earned high marks because he had begun his studies on the "best possible material for experiment—himself."[14] Chittenden then extended his dietary research to four of his colleagues, a detachment of men from the

Hospital Corps of the U.S. Army, and a group of college athletes. Antivivisectionists would perhaps have been less kind had they realized that four members of the army squad, disgruntled by the reduction to two-thirds of their normal military ration, were dropped from the study after devouring the free lunch at a nearby saloon.[15] But experiments on human volunteers, disgruntled or not, were more useful than those conducted on animals— the lack of species difference made the results directly applicable to humans— and the use of consenting subjects was considered to be less morally destructive to investigators than inflicting pain on helpless animals.

The establishment of the Rockefeller Institute for Medical Research, which opened its laboratories in 1904, contributed significantly to the groundswell of concern about animal experimentation. From the initial announcement of John D. Rockefeller's grant to establish a medical research institute, animal protectionists expressed alarm at a laboratory wholly devoted to vivisectional medicine and science. In 1907, when the Institute announced the purchase of a New Jersey farm for the production of laboratory animals, a reporter from the *New York Herald* (whose editor, James Gordon Bennett, opposed vivisection) forecast the coming storm over animal experimentation.[16] Subsequent developments justified his prediction. Two years later, when arsonists burned the farm, New Jersey authorities attributed the blaze to "unbalanced persons" whose judgment was affected by reports of vivisectors' cruelties.[17]

The growing prominence of the Rockefeller Institute for Medical Research fostered the organization of two new antivivisection societies in the New York area. The Society for the Prevention of Abuse in Animal Experimentation, established in 1907, and the New York Anti-Vivisection Society, organized in 1908, vigorously pursued the vivisection issue with the aid of several New York newspapers. Frederick Bellamy, legal counsel to the abuse prevention society, enlisted publisher William Randolph Hearst and his newspaper chain in the campaign against nontherapeutic human experimentation. The *New York Herald*, already feuding with members of the New York medical profession who opposed lucrative nostrum advertisements, joined the Hearst newspapers in attacking vivisectors.[18]

In February 1908 Diana Belais organized a public meeting at the Carnegie Lyceum to establish the New York Anti-Vivisection Society. Belais, whose husband was president of the New York Humane Society, recruited several celebrities, including two popular actresses, Minnie Maddern Fiske and Clara Morris, and the noted opera diva Emma Eames, and the meeting attracted considerable public attention.[19] Led by Belais, the New York Anti-

Vivisection Society consistently monitored the activities of the Rockefeller Institute. In addition to maintaining a small booth near the institute where they encouraged pet owners to seek their lost dogs and cats in the institute's animal house, members of the society induced one of the scrubwomen from the animal house, Mary Kennedy, to sign a complaint against the institute alleging cruelty to animals in the laboratory. Simon Flexner, the scientific director of the Institute, in turn swore out an affidavit denouncing an attempt by Kennedy to bribe other employees to lie about the conditions in the Rockefeller animal house. More damaging to Kennedy's credibility was an accusation by Flexner that she had tried to sell her neighbor's cat to the institute.[20] Concern about the growing criticism of the Rockefeller Institute's research may have directly benefited the research animals; the agitation led the institute's administrators to provide funds for a trained nurse to oversee the postoperative care of the animal subjects of Alexis Carrel's experiments in transplantation.[21]

The New York antivivisection societies also sought legislative solutions to the vivisection issue, pursuing laws to restrict the practice of animal experimentation in New York State. Each year from 1907 through 1923 one or more bills restricting animal experimentation appeared on the docket of the legislature. In 1908, when the *New York Medical Journal*, the *New York Times*, the *New York Evening Post*, and over seven hundred physicians from Brooklyn and New York City expressed support for legal regulation of animal experimentation, leaders of the American Medical Association formed a special committee to oppose such legislation. The Council on the Defense of Medical Research included Simon Flexner of the Rockefeller Institute, surgeon Harvey Cushing from Johns Hopkins, pharmacologist David L. Edsall from the University of Pennsylvania, and was headed by Walter Cannon, who was a physiologist at Harvard. The committee successfully persuaded the *New York Medical Journal* to rescind its initial backing of the antivivisection bill. Cannon subsequently engineered organized medicine's response to the antivivisectionists for the next eighteen years.[22]

The New York antivivisectionist organizations joined their colleagues in Philadelphia, Boston, Baltimore, and Washington, D.C., to create the Interstate Conference for the Investigation of Vivisection. Formed in 1912 to provide a national focus for their activities concerning animal and human experimentation, the conference received national exposure when the issue of human vivisection took center stage at its meeting in Washington, D.C., in December 1913.[23]

Human vivisection, especially the use of vulnerable children in non-

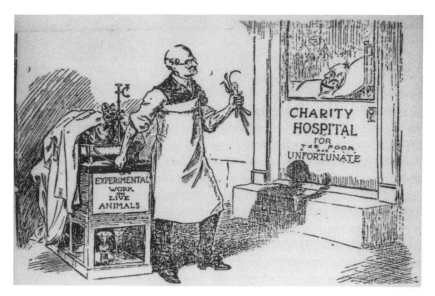

Cartoon entitled "Only a Step" illustrates one antivivisectionist view of the relationship between animal and human experimentation. New York *Herald*, reprinted in New York Anti-Vivisection Society pamphlet, 1914.

therapeutic experiments, was a favored target of Diana Belais and the New York Anti-Vivisection Society. Her campaign against human vivisection began in 1910 in *Cosmopolitan*, a popular Hearst magazine. Cruelty in animal experimentation, Belais argued, was closely related to the research exploitation of human beings. In both cases, the most vulnerable creatures became the subjects of experiments in which they could expect no benefit. In addition to the examples of nontherapeutic experimentation familiar to anyone who read the antivivisectionist press (Wentworth's lumbar punctures and Berkley's thyroid extract tests), Belais warned readers about a new danger, the growing number of clinical trials with tuberculin involving children in Philadelphia, New York, and Baltimore.[24]

In 1908 Samuel McClintock Hamill, Howard C. Carpenter, and Thomas A. Cope, pediatricians and associates of the William Pepper Clinical Laboratory at the University of Pennsylvania, reported the results of a study comparing three diagnostic tests for tuberculosis, named for their devisors. Each test involved the administration of tuberculin, the glycerinated extract of the tubercle bacillus that had initially been regarded as a cure for tuberculosis by Robert Koch. The Calmette test required the instillation of tuberculin solution into the eye, the Moro test the injection of tuberculin into the muscle, and the von Pirquet test injection of tuberculin into the skin. Hamill and his associates applied the tests to more than one hundred and sixty

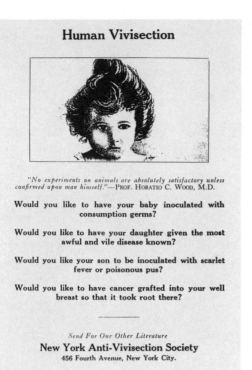

Human Vivisection

"No experiments on animals are absolutely satisfactory unless confirmed upon man himself."—Prof. Horatio C. Wood, M.D.

Would you like to have your baby inoculated with consumption germs?

Would you like to have your daughter given the most awful and vile disease known?

Would you like your son to be inoculated with scarlet fever or poisonous pus?

Would you like to have cancer grafted into your well breast so that it took root there?

Send For Our Other Literature

New York Anti-Vivisection Society
456 Fourth Avenue, New York City.

Excerpt from a pamphlet protesting human vivisection, published by the New York Anti-Vivisection Society, 1915.

children under the age of eight, all but twenty-six of whom resided in the St. Vincent's Home for Orphans, a Catholic orphanage in Philadelphia. Hamill concluded that the Calmette test, although easier to use, had serious disadvantages.[25] In their published report, the pediatricians described the discomforts and injuries that resulted from the eye test, including "a decidedly uncomfortable lesion" and "serious inflammations of the eye."[26]

Diana Belais emphasized the discomfort the young orphans experienced as a result of the tests, discomfort that bore no relation to their welfare. "The little children would lie in their beds moaning all night from the pain in their eyes," she somberly observed. "They kept their little hands pressed over their eyes, unable to sleep from the sensations they had to undergo."[27] She also provided names and photographs of Kitty Logan, "Little Catherine," and Agnes Morgan, the "material used" by Hamill and his colleagues.[28] The children at St. Vincent's were more vulnerable to "wicked exploitation" than the children at other Philadelphia child care institutions, speculated Jessica Henderson, another antivivisectionist, because the parents at day nurseries "would demand an explanation if their children were experimented upon and made to suffer."[29]

The clinical testing of tuberculin was not confined to Philadelphia.

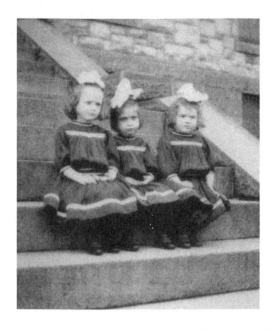

Illustration of "experimental material," from an exposé on the experimental use of orphans from St. Vincent's Home, Philadelphia. From "Vivisection Animal and Human," *Cosmopolitan*, 1910.

Belais also criticized the eminent New York pediatrician L. Emmett Holt's one thousand tuberculin tests on young children at Babies' Hospital in New York City.[30] In 1909 Holt, a professor of diseases of children at the Columbia University's College of Physicians and Surgeons, reported the results of his comparison of the ophthalmic tuberculin test and the von Pirquet skin test. Holt's "astonishing callousness" in describing tuberculin testing of "sick and dying babies" disgusted Belais and her colleagues, who challenged the therapeutic intentions of the physicians.[31]

Antivivisectionists emphasized the researchers' insensitivity to their young subjects. The American Anti-Vivisection Society and the Vivisection Investigation League issued identical pamphlets criticizing another comparative study of tuberculin testing, which appeared shortly after the reports of Holt and Hamill's group in Philadelphia. Both societies condemned the "callous and indifferent manner" in which Baltimore physicians Louis Hamman and Samuel Wolman referred to the "rich material at our disposal" at the Phipps Dispensary at Johns Hopkins Hospital.[32] Appalled by the repetition of a diagnostic test that involved permanent injury to children, antivivisectionists provided a lengthy list of physicians who rejected further use of the eye test, including Clemens von Pirquet, the respected Austrian pediatrician who devised the muscular injection test, and the AMA's Committee for Study of the Relation of Tuberculosis to Diseases of the Eye.[33] The pamphlets' compilers noted the committee's disapproval of the eye test, even though the committee's report did not altogether condemn the application of tuberculin to the eye.[34] For antivivisectionists, these multiple trials of tuberculin illustrated the extent to which experimentation, instead of resolving issues, generated more experimentation.

The development of a diagnostic test for syphilis, tested on orphans and hospital patients, further propelled the opposition to human vivisection. In 1911 Hideyo Noguchi, a microbiologist at the Rockefeller Institute for Medical Research, published the results of a promising series of experiments on rabbits and human beings with luetin, an inactive solution of *Treponema pallidum*, the causative agent of syphilis.[35] At the Rockefeller Institute syphilis was a major focus of study. Developments that led to a clearer understanding of the disease—namely, the identification of the spirochete in 1905, the development of the Wassermann blood test in 1906, and Paul Ehrlich's announcement of a specific curative drug (Salvarsan) for the disease in 1910—also fostered anticipation that the disease could be controlled and cured.[36] Noguchi believed that his success in growing pure cultures of the treponeme and the discovery of a specific skin reaction were critical steps in the search for a serum that would cure syphilis. He predicted that the luetin test would provide a useful complement to the Wassermann test, especially in diagnosing cases in the tertiary and congenital stages of the disease.

Inspired by Clemens von Pirquet's use of a skin test to diagnose tubercular infection, Noguchi hoped to develop an analogous test for the presence of the syphilitic organism. He had already performed a number of tests on animals to determine the safety and utility of the luetin test when William Henry Welch suggested that he make the test on human subjects. "Through his encouragement," Noguchi wrote, "I commenced the work at once at different dispensaries and hospitals with the cooperation of the physicians in charge."[37]

With the aid of fifteen physicians in the New York metropolitan area, Noguchi obtained four hundred subjects. Over half of the subjects had already been diagnosed as syphilitic or parasyphilitic. The remaining one hundred forty-six represented "various controls," including forty-six "normal" children between the ages of 2 and 18 and one hundred adults and children hospitalized for such nonsyphilitic diseases as malaria, leprosy, tuberculosis, and pneumonia.[38]

Noguchi's initial reports about luetin's utility caused considerable excitement in the United States and abroad. The Rockefeller Institute received numerous inquiries from physicians, including one request from the New York City Department of Health for enough luetin to perform 4,500 cutaneous injections.[39] Although the luetin test did not meet Noguchi's expectations, the initial interest and encouraging reports from physicians who tested luetin in their own practices prompted the institute to trademark the name and to license two pharmaceutical companies to produce and market the extract.[40]

Noguchi's use of normal children and hospital patients immediately attracted the censure of American antivivisectionists. In the spring of 1912 the two New York antivivisectionist societies issued circulars containing passages excerpted from Noguchi's paper in the *Journal of Experimental Medicine*, coupled with a warning about the dangers that unregulated experimentation posed for an unsuspecting public. The Vivisection Investigation League published an abbreviated account of the skin test for syphilis, which, without explicitly accusing Noguchi of infecting orphans with syphilis, implied that the inoculation of the dead germs of syphilis would certainly afflict the children. "Are the helpless people in our hospitals and asylums," the unnamed author asked, "to be treated as so much material for scientific experimentation, irrespective of age or consent?"[41] Throughout the protracted controversy, antivivisectionists continued to stress Noguchi's violation of the personal rights of the healthy children and ailing adults he had used in clinical trials of luetin.

Experiments with the syphilis germs, "one of the most loathsome diseases known to humanity," and Noguchi's affiliation with an institution devoted largely to vivisectional experimentation, made him an irresistible target of antivivisectionist animus.[42] Syphilis had only recently emerged from the "conspiracy of silence" that had enshrouded discussions of venereal disease during the Victorian era.[43] Public and medical attitudes toward syphilis and gonorrhea were changing in the second decade of the twentieth century; for the first time, the disease could be openly discussed in the pages of popular magazines and newspapers.[44] But venereal disease for many Americans remained a divine punishment for sins of the flesh. The idea that Noguchi deliberately introduced into the bodies of innocent children the germs—sterilized or not—of a loathsome disease repulsed many antivivisectionists, already suspicious of blood contamination and pollution.

In 1911 as part of the American Medical Association's Defense of Research Series, J. W. Churchman contributed an article on the advances in the study of syphilis resulting from animal experimentation.[45] When the *Journal of Zoophily* criticized the search for a cure for syphilis, William Keen wrote to Caroline Earle White for an explanation. "I cannot imagine," White informed Keen, "how the moral status of human beings can be anything but seriously impaired by the knowledge that they can with impunity give way to their evil passions, escaping the penalty imposed by God upon ill-doing."[46] Keen compared her response to the opposition that accompanied the introduction of anesthesia for women during childbirth. "The sad fact that many innocents suffered as a result of syphilitic infection," he argued, justified the medical search for a cure.[47] White, however, did not accept Keen's explanation and rejected altogether the use of "innocents" in experimental research directed toward discovering a cure to a disease intended to punish the guilty.

Noguchi's association with the Rockefeller Institute intensified antivivisectionists' misgivings. Any activity funded by John D. Rockefeller, the man Robert LaFollette called the "greatest criminal of our age," was likely to attract criticism. As the historian John Ettling has observed of Rockefeller, in his study of the Rockefeller Sanitary Commission, "perhaps no other American of his day was so despised."[48] Rockefeller's ruthless business methods and his enormous wealth created suspicion about all of his philanthropic efforts, including the creation of the Rockefeller Foundation. Only a selfish desire to extend his own life, observed one contributor to *Life,* could explain Rockefeller's interest in medical research—concern for human welfare was certainly not the explanation.[49]

Suspicion about Rockefeller's motive for establishing a hospital at the institute may also explain the trustees' decision to circulate a press release to New York newspapers announcing that experimentation on patients would not be undertaken. Amid charges of mistreatment and brutality involving indigent patients at three of the large city hospitals in New York City, the board in 1910 had announced, "It has been supposed that a hospital connected with an Institute for Medical Research would be one in which the patients were to be experimented upon, but the trustees wish it understood clearly that this is not the case."[50] The trustees were pleased by the outcome of this approach; the hospital received more than seventy requests from potential patients for treatment prior to the opening of the hospital and over two thousand applications for admission in the first four months of the hospital's operation.[51] The board's assurances notwithstanding, when antivivisectionists investigated Noguchi's experiments made a year later, they learned that he had used hospital patients in his tests.

For the most part, antivivisectionists directed little criticism at the Japanese physician himself, reserving their attacks for the American physicians who had collaborated with him. Noguchi's nationality may have insulated him from criticism; the "Oriental admirer of the fruits of Western civilization" successfully maintained a low public profile throughout the controversy over the luetin tests.[52] A trip to Europe in 1913 helped him avoid personal contact with his critics, as did the efforts of the business managers of the Rockefeller Institute. Although Sue M. Farrell, president of the Vivisection Investigation League, and Frederick Bellamy, counsel for the Society for the Prevention of Abuse in Animal Experimentation, persisted in their attempts to obtain interviews with Noguchi, in order to learn the names of his subjects, the institute's administrators apparently shielded Noguchi from encounters with antivivisectionists.

The brunt of criticism was borne by Noguchi's colleagues. William Henry Welch, well known in antivivisectionist circles for his effective opposition to legislative restrictions on animal experimentation, became a target, because it was he who had suggested that Noguchi test luetin on human beings. Antivivisectionists also condemned the lapse of "Judeo-Christian charity" on the part of the medical superintendents and hospital physicians whose "courtesy" had enabled Noguchi to conduct the trials with luetin. The American Anti-Vivisection Society, the New York Anti-Vivisection Society, and the Vivisection Investigation League, in their concern to identify Noguchi's "medical conspirators," published in full the names and hospital affiliations of the physicians who had provided Noguchi access to their wards.[53] "Courtesy is not, as a rule, alarming," the editor of *Life* characteristically observed,

> but the word takes on a new meaning when a Rockefeller scientist is permitted to experiment on 146 hospital patients through the "courtesy" of the physicians in charge. . . . If the researcher had said to these patients: "Have I your permission to inject into your system a concoction more or less related to a hideous disease?"—the invalids might have declined. The more courteous physicians, however, kindly grant permission to experiment—not on themselves—but on 146 human beings in their care.[54]

Antivivisectionists found the "professional etiquette" of experimenters particularly offensive. The often formulaic expressions of appreciation for the house physicians who gave investigators access to patients, a practice more common in the pediatric literature, struck many antivivisectionists as an ironic and dangerous development in the "esprit de corps of the medical profession."[55]

In the spring of 1912, when reports of Noguchi's luetin experiments involving children became public, Jerome D. Greene, business manager of the Rockefeller Institute, moved swiftly to neutralize antivivisectionist criticism. In an attempt to counter the charges of human vivisection, Greene provided Farrell with 350 reprints of Noguchi's article in the *Journal of Experimental Medicine*, together with a one-page statement he had prepared that recast "the language of the laboratory" into a more accessible account for lay readers.[56] Bacteriology was still a relatively new science, and the popular press was an active source of misinformation about it. Greene hoped to show that Noguchi's efforts to insure the sterility of luetin made it impossible for the inoculation to cause syphilis. The microscopic examination for evidence of live spirochetes, cultivation in artificial media, and inoculation into rabbits, Greene argued, demonstrated the safety of the extract. Moreover, Greene explained, Noguchi and several of his colleagues had first tested luetin on themselves to establish the safety of the test. Noguchi omitted this fact from his published papers, perhaps because of his own medical history: in 1913 doctors diagnosed his heart enlargement (aortic insufficency) as the result of an old, untreated syphilitic infection; he refused treatment for this condition at the Rockefeller Hospital.[57]

The references to control cases in the luetin trials needed careful handling. Greene admitted that, in an initial demonstration of a scientific procedure, some persons could legitimately be called controls. A diagnostic test is valuable to the extent that it reliably identifies disease; thus, testing on subjects known to be free of disease would be necessary to verify that the luetin test would give a negative result. But Greene argued that Noguchi's "so-called controls" actually benefited through their participation in the luetin testing. Although they were considered to be free of the disease, a positive response to the test enabled them to receive treatment for the disease for the first time.

The utility of such a test to hospitals impressed Greene. "What public institution," Greene asked, "would not welcome a harmless and painless test which would enable it to decide in the case of every person admitted whether that person was afflicted with a venereal disease or not?"[58] Greene did not address the issue of consent, the permission of guardians for the child participants, or any attempt to locate volunteers. In defense of Noguchi's "medical conspirators," Greene stressed the normal course of progress in medicine that required some individuals to serve as the initial recipients for new drugs or procedures, but only *after* animal experimentation had demonstrated their safety. Finally, Greene pointed to the success of the luetin test and its subsequent adoption in hospitals in Europe and America. The fact that luetin worked, he argued, tempered the negligible risk and slight discomfort some hospital patients had experienced in the initial demonstration of the test.

Despite Greene's efforts to defuse the controversy, in May 1912 John V. Lindsay, president of the New York Society for the Prevention of Cruelty to Children, instituted a formal complaint against Noguchi on charges of assault.[59] In a meeting with Greene and Assistant District Attorney James B. Reynolds, Lindsay argued that subjecting nonsyphilitic children to the luetin test without their consent or the consent of their legal guardians was technically illegal, although he acknowledged that the law regarding experimentation of this kind was not completely clear and that legislation might be required to clarify the issues. The Manhattan District Attorney's Office declined to prosecute Noguchi on criminal charges. Despite this vindication at the hands of the public prosecutor and despite acclaim of Noguchi by a number of New York newspapers, accusations of human vivisection continued to plague the Rockefeller staff.[60]

Pennsylvania legislator Henry Lanius, Caroline White, and other antivivisectionists supported procedures or innovative therapies that were expressly undertaken to benefit the patient. Indeed they preferred this approach to the less direct experiment on animals. They challenged the clinical testing of new and untried vaccines on hospital patients and institutionalized children, however. In 1913 concern about the Rockefeller experiments and the tuberculin testing at St. Vincent's Home encouraged the American Anti-Vivisection Society to support the introduction of a bill before the Pennsylvania legislature to regulate human experimentation. In his arguments in support of the proposal, Henry Lanius insisted that the bill did not interfere with research intended to benefit participants; its purpose was to prevent physicians from making experiments, procedures that had nothing to do with the patients' treatment: "By an experiment I mean the trying out of a theory by an operation. If a person was operated upon for some certain condition which existed, and the physician thought that the operation was going to relieve the patient, it does not come under this act because it is not an experiment. . . . If you seek to heal and cure, you are not experimenting."[61]

Although the bill to regulate human vivisection in Pennsylvania received the support of nearly one hundred legislators in at least two separate readings, it failed to pass. The physicians who traveled to Harrisburg to testify against the proposal successfully persuaded legislators that regulation would retard medical progress and inhibit the development of new medical therapies.[62]

The development of vaccines and other prophylactic measures created difficulties because they were intended to prevent disease that did not yet exist in a patient. (Moreover, many of the vaccines heralded in the press later proved to be worthless.) The moral questions were not new. The introduction of variolation against smallpox in the early eighteenth century prompted similar moral concerns about doing harm in the hope of helping someone avert a worse disease.[63]

In 1913 claims about a new tuberculosis vaccine aroused antivivisectionist concern for the welfare of children in a North Carolina orphanage. Karl von Ruck, who owned and operated a tuberculosis sanitarium in Asheville, had announced the successful immunization of 262 children from the nearby Baptist Orphanage, experiments made possible "through the interest and courtesy of Dr. C. A. Julian."[64] Impressed by early trials of the vaccine, the surgeon general of the U.S. Navy in 1913 had considered immunizing all soldiers and marines with the von Ruck vaccine, until a Senate-ordered investigation called into question the vaccine's safety and raised the possibility that it had actually increased the children's susceptibility to tuberculosis.[65] At the December 1913 meeting of the International Anti-Vivisection and Animal Protection Congress, von Ruck's experiments came under heavy attack, and "sensational" stories of vivisecting doctors appeared again in newspapers around the country.[66]

Yet von Ruck, who continued to maintain the value of his vaccine, denied that his tests on orphans constituted experimentation. "The work done at the Baptist Orphanage," he privately informed William Keen, "was, under no circumstances, an experiment but it was based on ample experience with both the old and the new vaccine. The only question was, whether we could immunize with a single dose instead of many."[67] Von Ruck's references in his published papers to experiments on children did not help his case, but they illustrate the ambiguity about what constituted an experiment and what could be considered legitimate, if innovative, treatment. Von Ruck did not undertake the experiment that would have definitively established the value of his vaccine. Unlike the early nineteenth-century physicians who challenged vaccination with injections of smallpox matter to see whether children would develop smallpox, von Ruck did not inject the children who received his vaccine with live tubercle bacilli to see whether they became tuberculous. "Such an experiment," noted A. M. Stimson, the Public Health Service investigator sent to evaluate von Ruck's research, "is obviously impossible."[68]

Using orphans in trials of the vaccine was sufficient to arouse antivivisectionists. Attorney Frank Stephens branded von Ruck's experiments "worse than the slaughter of the innocents." Unfortunately, it was not his only new example of child vivisection. Stephens described injections with the germs of bovine and human tuberculosis into "nine charity children" from the Washington Children's Hospital in 1908, the experimental inoculation of previously uninfected children with ringworm, as well as Noguchi's luetin tests on orphans and hospital patients.[69]

The growing number of cases persuaded Senator Gallinger to sponsor a bill in 1914 calling for a formal commission to investigate charges that human beings were being used as subjects in nontherapeutic experiments in public hospitals. Similar proposals were introduced in the state legislatures of New York and New Jersey.[70] The Hearst newspapers supported these proposals and continued to print stories of patients' being used in scientific research without their consent. In New York City, where clamor over human vivisection was the greatest, several anxious parents appealed to the Vivisection Investigation League for information to help them determine whether their children had been subjected to involuntary nontherapeutic experiments.[71] Several individuals instituted civil suits against New York hospitals for allegedly infecting their children with venereal disease.[72] Reports that young children hospitalized for treatment of such contagious diseases as measles and scarlet fever received experimental inoculations of syphilis prompted an investigation of forty-eight children allegedly infected in two Bronx hospitals. The Bronx district attorney, the New York City Department of Health, and the New York Commission of Charities conducted investigations of the charges against the Riverside and Willard Parker hospital staffs. Interviews with twenty-five families involving thirty-four children revealed that none of the children had syphilis, nor had any of the children received serum or vaccine inoculations during their hospitalizations.[73] The health commissioner conceded that some of the girls suffered from gonorrheal vaginitis, an apparently common disease among children in New York City.[74]

The collapse of the charges against the Bronx hospitals and the failure to demonstrate that Noguchi or any other physician had harmed their hospital patients prompted sharp criticism of Hearst and the New York antivivisectionists. "The Hearst newspapers are read largely by the poor and ignorant, who are afraid of authority wherever they find it, and who already

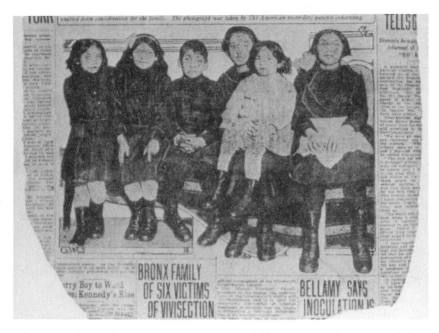

Photograph illustrating a newspaper report that children had been intentionally infected with disease while at the hospital seeking other treatment. "Bronx Family of Six Victims of Vivisection," *New York American*, 16 February 1914.

have a deep-rooted prejudice against the medical profession," wrote one critic. "Whenever Hearst indulges in a scare of this sort, not only is the work of preventive medicine retarded, but cases of contagious diseases are concealed from the doctors. Frightened mothers refrain from taking their sick babies to the hospital."[75] This criticism did little to deter antivivisectionist attacks on the abuse of patients' rights in human vivisection. The New York Anti-Vivisection Society, for example, solicited physician opinions about the human vivisections at the Rockefeller Hospital.[76]

The continuing allegations about Noguchi's luetin test inspired the Rockefeller staff to consider filing a libel suit against the antivivisectionists. Although encouraged by English cases in which medical researchers had won damages when maliciously inaccurate descriptions of their work appeared in print, the institute staff eventually rejected such a step as "unwise."[77] Their legal advisers warned that libel cases were difficult to win; a successful legal action required a convincing demonstration of the actual material harm caused by the libel.[78] The decision to forgo a suit also reflected the ambiguous ethical and legal status of human experimentation during this period.

Jerome Greene and several of his colleagues believed that the seed of the controversy over the luetin experiments was indiscriminate use of the word *control* and the unfortunate image it conveyed to a lay reader: "To an anti-vivisectionist, the word naturally conjures up pictures of human vivisection in which normal human beings have experiments made on them as a means of checking experiments on diseased human beings. The situation is sufficiently delicate to necessitate very careful handling."[79] Although persuaded that the prior testing of luetin on animals and physician-volunteers cleared Noguchi of the charge of human vivisection, Greene and other members of the Rockefeller staff acknowledged that the legal situation concerning the consent of the children and adults tested in hospitals was ambiguous.

This did not prevent Greene from taking a hard line with the president of the Vivisection Investigation League. He rebuked Sue Farrell for making the gratuitous assumption that Noguchi had violated the individual rights of his subjects. "It does not seem reasonable to expect," Greene informed her, "that a high-minded and humane investigator should accompany every description of a scientific procedure with a declaration that he acted with a due regard to the rights of all persons concerned."[80] Although Greene insisted that consent of the healthy subjects had been attended to, it seems unlikely that Noguchi had in fact consulted his subjects for their permission to participate; he did not acknowledge their cooperation in his papers. Henry James, Jr., who succeeded Greene as business manager of the institute, apparently did not share his predecessor's perception of this aspect of the luetin affair. James conceded the technical impropriety of Noguchi's luetin tests: "Noguchi took liberties if you like, but he did nothing dangerous. His wrong is what lawyers call 'a wrong without injury.' "[81] James did not treat the technical violation of the rights of the children and hospital patients as a serious infraction.

The legal question of consent again arose when the institute staff considered bringing a suit against Frank Stephens, the attorney who had maligned Noguchi's experiments at the 1913 International Anti-Vivisection and Animal Protection Congress. Talking with Martin Cohen, a physician associated with the Randall's Island Asylum and the chief source of Noguchi's child subjects, made James reluctant to press a civil suit against Stephens. Cohen, like Noguchi, had himself voluntarily undergone the luetin test and then allowed Noguchi to apply the test to the children in his charge. He acknowledged to James that the children were all wards of the New York Board of Charities, whose authority was required for even "an unnecessary pinprick." If the Board of Charities had approved the tests, no one admitted that fact.

Uncertainty about the legal status of experimentation on the children in Cohen's care led James to inform Rockefeller attorney Starr J. Murphy, "Although I think that the issues could be limited so that the testimony as to the consent of the 'controls' could be kept out of the case, this is a point about which you rightly observe that we could not be absolutely certain."[82] In James's opinion, Noguchi would not be held liable for the experiments; rather, the responsibility lay with Cohen and the other physicians who had supplied Noguchi's subjects. James decided that when a libel suit against an antivivisectionist was inevitably splashed all over the pages of the Hearst newspapers, maintaining such distinctions would be difficult, especially after Cohen became the target of antivivisectionist attack.[83]

The controversy over the luetin trial spurred James to give greater scrutiny to written materials that could be misunderstood by a lay audience—and in the case of antivivisectionists, a hostile one. The business manager advised the pharmaceutical company H. K. Mulford to avoid using such terms as *controls* and *human material* in its advertising circular for the syphilis test. James offered the firm explicit directions, suggesting that, in the discussion of the initial tests of luetin, Mulford delete the description of the controls as "50 non-syphilitic children and 200 adults suffering from various diseases" and insert instead the phrase "numerous cases of tuberculosis, leprosy, etc."[84]

The leaders of the defense of medical research hoped to avert any drop in public regard for the medical research community. Walter Bradford Cannon, who continued to coordinate organized medicine's response to antivivisection, developed several strategies to counteract accusations made against physicians who experimented on hospital patients. First he explicitly confronted the issue of human vivisection in a series of pamphlets organized to educate physicians about the benefits of animal experimentation. He then turned to his extensive network of physicians supportive of research and asked them to investigate the individual experimenters charged with improper human experimentation.

Cannon recruited Richard Mills Pearce, a physiologist at the University of Pennsylvania, to write the only pamphlet about human vivisection in the Defense of Research Series. His article, which appeared in February 1914, during the height of the Hearst campaign over "babies, blood, and science" accused antivivisectionists not only of malicious misrepresentation in discussions of human vivisection but of cooperating with "forces opposed to the improvement of public health."[85] Pearce was familiar with antivivisectionist attacks. At the time his pamphlet appeared, he was scheduled to appear in a Philadelphia court with four colleagues from the physiology department on charges of cruelty to animals.[86]

Pearce challenged antivivisectionist reports of serious injury resulting from Berkley's use of thyroid tablets and Wentworth's lumbar punctures. He conceded the unfortunate character of two experiments on humans: Stickler's injection of children with the germs of foot-and-mouth disease in 1887 and the attempts by "crank" physician M. J. Rodermund to disprove the germ theory of disease. Stickler and Rodermund, Pearce argued, were hardly representative of the medical profession. Pearce explained that Stickler had been of unsound mind when he made his experiments on children, saying that Stickler's suicide confirmed his friends' impression that he was "mentally unbalanced for a time—obsessed that he was immortalizing his name and would deserve the gratitude of future generations."[87]

Unlike Stickler, who had graduated from Columbia's College of Physicians and Surgeons, Rodermund was labeled a "crank" and a "pseudoscientist" for his refusal to accept the theory that germs caused disease.[88] Rodermund claimed that, after having conducted several animal experiments, he sprayed the poisons of smallpox, diphtheria, scarlet fever, and consumption into the throats of seventeen people between the ages of 15 and 30, explaining, "Of course, I could not let the patients know what I was doing. I was supposed to be treating them for catarrh of the nose or throat."[89] Rodermund concluded that the failure of his patients to develop these diseases disproved the germ theory. In another flamboyant demonstration of his belief that contagion was "a medical superstition," Rodermund smeared his own body with "smallpox pus," which led to his involuntary incarceration in a Milwaukee infectious disease hospital.[90]

Pearce benefited from private information about Rodermund provided by Cannon, who monitored incidents that could be used against the medical profession for the purpose of curtailing laboratory freedom. Cannon had written to several physicians in Wisconsin, where Rodermund practiced, exploring the possibility that Rodermund's medical license could be revoked. Both Joseph Erlanger, a University of Wisconsin physiologist, and J. L. Yates, a Milwaukee physician, assured Cannon in 1909 that Rodermund was a "fake" with no standing in the community.[91] Despite some misgivings about allowing Rodermund to continue to practice medicine, neither Cannon nor the Wisconsin Medical Society intervened, however. Nearly a year after their exchange, Yates sent Cannon a newspaper clipping describing how Rodermund had been charged with arson for setting his own office on fire.[92]

Pearce explained that, unlike Rodermund, Noguchi had followed the appropriate steps for extending medical knowledge. After first demonstrating the safety and efficacy of the luetin test on animals, Noguchi had experimented on himself and other physicians before applying the test to patients: "in these first crucial tests on man the greatest caution is observed and it is usually the investigator himself who submits to the test."[93] Following this act of heroism, patients received the preparation.

Pearce suggested that greater attention to the wording of published reports of clinical experiments on human beings would lessen criticism. He proposed that editors of medical journals be as careful of potential pitfalls in reporting clinical experiments with human beings as they were in describing the details of anesthesia and postoperative care in papers describing experiments on animals.[94] Similar proposals had followed the controversy over human vivisection at the turn of the century: in order to prevent "a chance for certain individuals to misconstrue facts and misrepresent and slander our profession," editors of the *Journal of the American Medical Association* had then recommended that colleagues exercise good judgment in reporting the results of human experiments.[95] A 1901 paper in the *Medical Record*, for example, described an experiment in surgical disinfection for which a human subject contributed finger scrapings. The reference to the subject as "our victim" was just the sort of sarcastic word play that alarmed defenders of medical research.[96] Not only professional papers but also advertisements came under scrutiny. In 1914 Walter Cannon criticized a Lederle advertisement for vaccine virus that boasted that the virus had been "physiologically tested on children," but gave no indication that the tests had proceeded with the permission of the parents or had benefited the children involved.[97] When the *Journal of the American Medical Association* included an editorial praising the experimental feeding of different types of pathogenic amebas to human beings, there was a similar lamentation about the potential for misunderstanding, this time from William Keen.[98]

In May 1914 in his capacity as chair of the Council on the Defense of Medical Research, Walter Cannon circulated among editors of medical journals a letter asking that original papers submitted for publication be edited to eliminate expressions that could be misunderstood by antivivisectionists and the public: "In any case of diagnosis or treatment when the procedure is novel or might be objected to, let the fact be stated that the patient or his family were fully aware of and consented to the plan."[99] Although Cannon received a number of letters from editors of medical journals who promised to adopt these suggestions, the problems of language remained.[100]

Cannon expressed surprise and anger when this advice was not heeded at the Rockefeller Institute. In February 1916 the *Journal of Experimental Medicine*, edited by Simon Flexner (who also served on Cannon's protection of medical research committee), published an article by a young professor of dermatology and syphilology at the University of Michigan Medical School. Udo Julius Wile reported his successful inoculation of rabbits with syphilitic treponemes obtained from the brains of patients in a Michigan mental institution.[101] This report sparked renewed concern, both public and professional, about the use of hospital patients in nontherapeutic research.

Following his graduation from the Johns Hopkins University Medical School in 1907, Udo Wile pursued postgraduate work in dermatological clinics in Europe.[102] In Berlin, he assisted in the research of two German investigators who performed brain punctures on patients with neurosyphilis in order to demonstrate the presence in life of active spirochetes in the brain tissues. Wile considered Edmund Forster and Egon Tomaszczewski's work especially significant because the presence of active spirochetes suggested that antisyphilitic drugs might be effective if introduced directly into the brain tissues.[103]

The possibility of early and effective treatment for a disease many physicians considered hopeless impressed Wile as needing further research. Although most investigators confined their studies to spirochetes obtained from the brain at autopsy, Wile argued that organisms obtained from living brains would be more useful for resolving the questions about a distinctive, neurotropic strain of syphilis.[104] He decided to repeat the brain punctures he had observed in Berlin on patients in the Pontiac State Hospital. In 1915 he chose six individuals with general paralysis whose diagnosis was based on clinical findings and positive Wassermann tests.[105]

According to Wile, the operation of brain puncture was extremely simple and painless. After the head of the patient was shaved and an anesthetic was applied to numb the area, Wile employed a revolving dental drill to pierce the skin and deeper tissues over the frontal convolution: "A few rapid revolutions of the drill in the hands of an assistant suffice to pierce the skull."[106] Wile then inserted a long, thin trocar needle into the hole and aspirated a small cylinder of brain substance. He explained that the procedure entailed few risks, though the operator of course needed to avoid the cerebral and meningeal arteries and to maintain sterile conditions.

In March 1916 antivivisectionists learned of Wile's brain punctures. The Vivisection Investigation League quickly issued a pamphlet warning that vivisection as a system had become so entrenched that physicians dared to publish openly the details of nontherapeutic experiments on hospital patients.[107] Stressing the question of risk, the possibility of pain, and disregard for the patient's rights, the compiler criticized the Rockefeller Institute and its director, Simon Flexner, for publishing Wile's paper without discussing its ethical shortcomings. In light of the Rockefeller Institute's involvement in another experiment with the germs of syphilis, the League demanded to know "how far this use of patients in our hospitals for purely experimental purposes will extend before public feeling is sufficiently aroused to take action?"[108]

Vehement antivivisectionist criticism kept the story active, and soon accounts of Wile's "dental drill experiments" appeared in newspapers around the country.[109] Antivivisectionists took comfort in the fact that Wile's experiments had at last aroused indignation on the part of many newspaper editors, who had previously supported the organized medical profession in the protection of medical research. *Living Tissue*, the magazine of the New England Anti-Vivisection Society, observed with obvious relish that the Baltimore *American*, the Philadelphia *Inquirer*, the New York *World*, and the Philadelphia *Bulletin* all had taken strong stands against the vivisection of human beings.[110]

Newspaper stories, however, included statements from physicians and surgeons who dismissed the idea that consent for harmless, nontherapeutic experiments was necessary. Several of the doctors quoted in newspapers insisted that admission to the hospital implied permission for any experiment deemed necessary by the physician. "The consent of the guardians or relatives of the patients was not secured as it was not necessary," the head of the Pontiac State Hospital stoutly maintained. Obtaining permission from such hopelessly diseased individuals as Wile's paretic patients was also unnecessary: "Paresis was inevitably taking those patients away, and the operation did not retard or hasten the course of the disease."[111] Wile, too, seemed indifferent to the published accounts of his operations on insane patients: "You may quote me as having absolutely no interest in the matter," Wile informed a reporter, "whatever people may wish to think regarding the experiment."[112]

Wile's apparent insensitivity to public opinion alarmed William Keen and Walter Bradford Cannon. They consulted Henry James, Jr., and Simon Flexner about the Rockefeller Institute's position on the Wile experiments. At the institute, publication of the Wile paper was considered a regrettable lapse of judgment. Flexner informed Keen that the manuscript had been accepted while he was out of the country, but the person responsible in Flexner's absence for its acceptance was not named.[113] James declared it impossible for anyone connected with the institute to address the Wile case in public, whether in support or condemnation of it, but he encouraged Keen and Cannon to take whatever steps seemed necessary to counteract the unfortunate impression of human vivisection. Observing that many members of the medical profession looked to their leadership, James insisted: "It is surely more important for you to maintain your position correctly, than it is to hush up the attacks on Wile. . . . Nothing could be more fatal to the defense of research in the long run than an unvarying, thick-and-thin defense by you and others of all doctors attacked by the Press."[114] In James's estimation, Wile clearly had overstepped the boundary of acceptable use of human beings in nontherapeutic experimentation. But, as in the case of Noguchi, James assigned the legal responsibility to the medical superintendent who had supplied Wile's subjects rather than to the investigator.

Although the Rockefeller staff declined public comment, Cannon and Keen believed that some action was necessary. Cannon disapproved of Wile's use of insane patients, but he hesitated to criticize the brain punctures openly for fear of lending substance to antivivisectionist attacks on human vivisection.[115] Publicly, Cannon chose to prepare an editorial for the *Journal of the American Medical Association* in April 1916 that expressed the "right and wrong of making experiments on human beings," but did not explicitly identify Wile. Privately, Cannon harshly informed the young Michigan physician that "no one man has any reason whatever to be disregardful of the conviction which mankind cherishes that the right of the individual to determine the uses to which his body shall be put, is a sacred right which no investigator is justified in violating." He pointed out that an experimenter who ignored public feeling about the limits of experimentation not only harmed himself but placed "in great danger the freedom of research which had been enjoyed in this country up to this time—a freedom which has had important values for the progress of medicine."[116]

The desire to clarify the relationship between clinical investigators and their patients encouraged Cannon to propose that the AMA amend its code of ethics to include a statement about the necessity of patient cooperation in experimentation.[117] The AMA's code of ethics, initially adopted in 1847 (and periodically revised), did not explicitly address the use of human subjects in research. Like the Hippocratic Oath and the English physician Thomas Percival's 1803 code on which it was modeled, the AMA's code of ethics focused on the physician's responsibilities to patients at the bedside and in the consulting room. It did not include, until 1946, the obligations of a researcher to a subject.

Cannon's 1916 recommendation that the AMA adopt a formal resolution on acceptable human experimentation troubled many of his colleagues leading the defense of research. Although such a resolution would have had little effect on the daily lives of most medical practitioners, physicians at elite institutions would presumably be affected by formal guidelines for clinical research. Henry James, Jr., conceded that an official stand on the subject was necessary: "many medical men are really in danger of supposing any harmless operation on a patient is justifiable if performed with a scientific purpose, even though the patient doesn't consent. I have heard this argued by most reputable and high-minded M.D.'s, but of course this view is one which is directly contrary to the law, and the lay public would never subscribe to it or tolerate asylum or University officers who encourage it."[118] James worried about where to draw the line between unjustifiable experiments on human beings and those procedures that, although unrelated to an individual's treatment, contributed significantly to clinical research. He hesitated to interfere with the routine hospital collections of such body fluids as blood, cerebrospinal fluid, and urine, or the taking of cardiographic information, because any interference with this work would slow the rate of progress in clinical research.

Other members of the Rockefeller staff shared James's views. Both Simon Flexner and Rufus Cole, director of the Rockefeller Hospital, expressed concern that "laboratory men" did not fully appreciate the point of view of the clinicians.[119] Flexner suggested that no rash action be taken; Cole preferred to see nothing done. Cole explained privately to Francis Peabody, a Boston physician, that he feared allowing the human experimentation resolution to come before the AMA delegates because it would "open the way for a discussion of the importance of obtaining the consent of the patient before any investigations are carried on which are not primarily for the welfare of the patient."[120] Drawing up guidelines for human experimentation, Cole contended, was not at all analogous to developing rules for carrying out experiments on dogs. While Cannon insisted on changing the code of ethics "to strengthen the hands of those who are resisting the antivivisectionists," Cole suggested that a "safer" approach would be to state: "In studying by new devices disease of human beings, or in testing a new diagnostic or curative method, the physician should regard the welfare of the patient as of primary importance. Before being applied, any new procedure should, if possible, be shown by experiments on lower animals to be free from danger to the patient."[121] Cole did not include patient consent in his proposed revision of the code.

Obtaining the formal and prior consent of a patient for every procedure conducted on a hospital ward struck Francis Peabody as unnecessary. In many cases, the cooperation of the patient constituted effective consent, he argued. "In practical work in medical wards," he informed Cannon, "the patients do virtually give their consent to what is done to them, and if they raise any objection the procedure is not carried out."[122] Peabody did feel that procedures involving surgery, anesthesia, or which were liable to injure the patient required physicians to obtain a patient's formal consent. The critical safeguard for patient welfare, he suggested, was not an explicit guideline for experimentation and the formal consent of the patient but the character of the clinical researcher. The individuals who pursued a career in scientific medicine, he believed, were generally "among the more high-minded of the profession."[123]

Despite Cannon's recommendation that there be a formal resolution stating the importance of obtaining patient consent and cooperation in experimentation, the American Medical Association's House of Delegates did not entertain his proposal at their meeting in 1916. Discussions about compulsory health insurance and issues related to the war in Europe occupied the delegates. (Although America did not formally enter the war until 1917, American physicians were already aiding the war effort by helping to organize military hospitals to care for wounded soldiers.)

The AMA did enable Cannon and William Keen to go on record against using patients in scientific experiments without their consent. Keen insisted that Wile's case demanded explicit condemnation; a failure of the medical profession to criticize Wile would justify antivivisectionist claims about medical indifference to human vivisection.[124] Although convinced that the brain punctures deserved condemnation, Keen nonetheless worried that his comments would play into the hands of antivivisectionists. He prepared a short critical statement, which he circulated among such leaders of medical research as Simon Flexner, Walter Cannon, Frederic Schiller Lee, Hans Zinsser, Victor C. Vaughan, William Welch, and Rufus Cole. His statement underwent considerable revision; even the title was changed from "Human Vivisection—A Protest" to "The Inveracities of Antivivisection." Keen was well pleased with the editorial changes, boasting to one of his colleagues that the revisions not only allowed him to go on record against Wile's research but to blunt the criticism with an attack on antivivisection and distortion.[125]

Keen's statement appeared in the November 4th issue of the *Journal of the American Medical Association*, together with Walter Cannon's editorial on the ethics of human experimentation.[126] In his remarks, Cannon outlined the physician's obligation to heal the sick, to check disease, and to prevent death. He also invoked the physician's obligation to advance medical progress. Acknowledging that devotion to learning occasionally tempted researchers to perform procedures without careful consideration of the rights of individual patients, Cannon observed: "There is no more primitive and fundamental right which any individual possesses than that of controlling the uses to which his own body is put. Mankind has struggled for centuries for the recognition of this right. Civilized society is based on the recognition of it. The lay public is perfectly clear about it."[127] Physicians and hospital administrators who countenanced such abuses, Cannon sternly warned, would suffer public hostility and legal action.

Yet the issues were far from clear. Physicians agreed that patient welfare was the chief responsibility of the medical profession but they differed about what constituted an experiment and over the value and meaning of patient consent. The search for new vaccines and diagnostic tests for infectious diseases raised questions about the definition of medical experimentation and about where to draw the line between an experimental procedure and an acceptable clinical practice. For practicing clinicians like Francis Peabody and Rufus Cole, the patient's cooperation in medical treatment implied authorization for research, so long as the research did not compromise the welfare of the patient. Introducing a requirement that physicians obtain explicit permission for research struck investigators as not only unnecessary but potentially damaging to the entire research enterprise. They preferred to ride out the storm of antivivisectionist criticism than risk interfering with medical progress and professional prerogative.

Chapter Five

"Your Dog and Your Baby":
The Continuing Campaign against
Human Vivisection

After 1916 American antivivisectionists maintained their opposition to the use of vulnerable human beings in medical research. As part of the ongoing campaign against animal experimentation, they continued to criticize experiments involving orphans, prisoners, and soldiers. Although the movement lost public support in the decade after World War I, emphasis on protecting pet animals—dogs and cats—from medical researchers contributed to a resurgence in antivivisectionist activity during the 1930s and prompted an influential segment of the research community to heed stories of laboratory abuse, animal and human.

Human vivisection remained an essential feature of the critique of animal experimentation. Rejecting claims that research on animals was necessary in order to prevent experimentation on human beings, antivivisectionists insisted that "It is NOT a question of Your Dog or Your Baby, but one of Your Dog AND Your Baby. It is not a question of animals or human beings, but one of animals AND human beings."[1] Some human beings were more vulnerable than others to experimenters. Like dogs and cats, infants and orphans were unable to protect themselves from ambitious investigators. Antivivisectionists devoted most of their attention to the children who participated in medical experiments or in trials of new vaccines.

To the "incurable injustice of experimentation upon infancy that can offer no protest but a cry," antivivisectionists added the exploitation of prisoners, soldiers, and even those adults who received compensation for their participation.[2] What united this diverse group of human subjects was their vulnerability. The constraints of military service and penal institutions made soldiers and prisoners available to serve as research subjects, but antivivisectionists were skeptical that these subjects were truly volunteers in research. Although paying men and women for their services as research subjects presumably insured awareness about a medical experiment, antivivisectionists questioned whether these individuals fully understood the risks and discomfort they would incur from participation.

This chapter explores some of the antivivisectionist objections to experiments involving children, soldiers, prisoners, and professional subjects in the years between the world wars. Although critics of animal experimentation concentrated on only a fraction of the growing number of experiments involving human subjects, these cases illustrate some of the problematic features of human experimentation before World War II. Enrolling orphans in clinical trials, for example, raised difficult questions about consent and guardianship. The use of prisoners invoked the potential for coercion. The antivivisectionist critique of research involving these populations prompted some medical researchers to consider strategies to diminish concerns about exploitation and coercion. Using written consent forms and compensation schemes and obtaining parental permission helped to ease anxieties—both professional and public—about experimental abuse. Defenders of medical research also successfully undermined charges of human vivisection by invoking the heroism of doctors who sacrificed themselves for medical science.

The outbreak of war in 1914 presaged a decline in public support for the American antivivisection movement. Even before America's entry into the war in 1917, antivivisectionists' opposition to typhoid vaccination for soldiers and their resistance to using animals to answer military medical questions created resentment. "Apparently in the presence of the enormous catastrophe in Europe where nations are thinking that the sacrifice of human life for national welfare is fully justified," Walter Bradford Cannon observed in 1915, "the 'Antis' find some difficulty in convincing people that it is wicked to use the lives of a relatively small number of lower animals for the welfare of all mankind as well as the animals themselves."[3] Crippled by the loss of leading activists (Caroline Earle White and Albert Leffingwell died in 1916) and influential supporters (Senator Jacob Gallinger died in 1918), the movement won few friends when they opposed a plan by the National Red Cross to fund animal experiments for research on trench fever.[4] When the U.S. War Department asked the Red Cross in 1917 to appropriate $100,000 for investigations into the nature and prevention of the disease plaguing the troops, antivivisectionists, with the support of the *Christian Science Monitor*, successfully blocked the use of general funds for the purpose. Although the Red Cross created a special fund for the trench fever project, antivivisection societies and Christian Scientists were roundly criticized for placing animal welfare before the needs of American soldiers.[5]

In the 1920s, the fortunes of the antivivisection movement continued to decline. Although some researchers feared that the extension of suffrage to women would doom medical freedom, the potential threat to animal experimentation failed to materialize. "The women of the country," observed Cornelia James Cannon in 1922, disproved "the accusation of sentimentality and over-emotionalism, made by those who were unwilling to admit them to full citizenship" by helping to defeat statewide measures to abolish animal experimentation in California (1920) and Colorado (1922).[6] Cornelia Cannon was hardly an unprejudiced observer; her husband Walter had been actively defending animal experimentation since 1908. But the legislative defeats, together with the impressive discovery of insulin achieved by research involving dogs, prompted some medical scientists to predict the imminent demise of the antivivisection movement. Antivivisection, crowed elder statesman of medicine William Henry Welch in 1926, "is a lost cause and the position of the adherents pathetic."[7]

Welch celebrated too soon. In the 1930s the movement rebounded with surprising readiness. Focusing on protecting pets from research helped the movement gain lost ground in only a few years. Membership in antivivisection societies rose sharply. The New England Anti-Vivisection Society, for example, listed 534 members in 1933; by 1944, the number of members had grown to nearly 5,000.[8] Renewed efforts at the federal, state, and local levels to restrict animal experimentation prompted the research community to reorganize its defense of medical research in order to avert legal regulations of laboratory animal use.[9]

The issue of human vivisection also played a role in reanimating the antivivisection movement. Attacks on the use of prisoners, soldiers, professional subjects, and, above all, orphans attracted public attention and created concern in the research community. Children received most of the attention of animal protectionists. Experiments on children raised problematic issues about consent, voluntariness, and parental responsibility. What did it mean to describe a child as a volunteer? Were infants and children only volunteers in the sense that some adults had "volunteered" them? Was it appropriate for parents to give consent for their children to participate in research when no benefit for the child was anticipated? In the case of orphans, who should be consulted to obtain permission for their participation in research? Although many Americans may have conceded the importance of medical research into childhood diseases, they understandably balked at using their own children as research subjects. Many others flinched at the research use of the most defenseless children, orphans. These unresolved tensions helped to make experiments involving orphans and hospitalized children a sensitive issue during the 1920s and 1930s.

Some physicians sought to minimize the legal and ethical problems raised by experiments on children by obtaining consent from parents for a child's participation and publishing that fact in the research paper. By securing a parent's permission to test a new vaccine or drug on a child, physicians may have hoped to avoid legal tangles in the event of a bad outcome. Parental permission may also have served to assuage a doctor's anxiety about harming a child. In the years between the world wars, a number of physicians reported that they had received parental permission before attempting novel treatments or using vaccines on children. In 1915, for example, Charles Hermann "obtained the consent of a mother to inoculate her infant" with measles virus collected on cotton swabs from the nose of an infected patient.[10] Although the New York pediatrician went on to inoculate thirty-nine other infants, he explained neither how he went about the securing of parental consent nor what the parents actually understood about the risks and benefits of his vaccine. Physicians acknowledged that being well-respected in the community helped them to persuade parents to allow their child's participation. When doctors Claud Johnson and Ernest Goodpasture sought to establish the etiology of mumps, a common childhood disease, they obtained permission from parents to infect seventeen children under experimental conditions in Johnson's home community, where he "was intimately known by those whose consent was obtained." The physician's standing in the community, as well as their familiarity with the usual outcome of mumps, influenced parents to authorize their children to participate. Nine of the seventeen "volunteers," aged three to twelve, developed the disease; happily, all recovered.[11]

Experimenting on one's own children made the formality of parental consent unnecessary, even as it raised other issues about the nature of parental responsibility. Although the children of physicians had long served as guinea pigs for their fathers—in the early trials of smallpox variolation and vaccination, for example—such experimentation had prompted little criticism.[12] In the 1930s, antivivisectionists challenged this traditional prerogative. In 1933, in order to verify the safety and efficacy of a newly developed whooping cough vaccine, pediatricians Hugh and E. J. MacDonald used their four sons as subjects. According to popular journalist Paul de Kruif, the

MacDonalds vaccinated two of their children with pertussis vaccine and then "sprayed whooping cough microbes into the noses of all of them."[13] The two "vaccinated volunteers" (ages 9 and 8) remained free of whooping cough, but the 6-year-old twins developed the severe coughs, paroxysms, and whoops symptomatic of the disease.[14] Antivivisectionists criticized these "unnatural parents" for subjecting their own children to a potentially dangerous disease to resolve a scientific question. Rather than endanger their children, mothers and fathers were expected to preserve the health and welfare of their children. For antivivisectionists, the MacDonald experiment provided yet another example of the vulnerability of children—even the offspring of physicians—and of the corrupting power of scientific ambition.

References to child participants as "volunteers" appeared frequently in medical papers. What the term actually meant to investigators, parents, or the children themselves is difficult to infer from these texts. The Mac-Donalds, for example, identified their sons as volunteers, but whether the boys understood the experiment or even cooperated with their parents remains unknown. The account of researcher Leon Goldman suggests that not all experiments on the children of doctors proceeded smoothly. Goldman's son apparently complained to his teachers that "his father forced him to put his arm in a cage with yellow-fever mosquitoes."[15] Because children lacked the ability to consent in meaningful ways to requests to participate in research or to undertake a particular therapy, antivivisectionists were offended by references to children as volunteers. When three Japanese investigators reported that they had experimentally produced scarlet fever in "volunteers" aged 3 to 7 years, one critic disputed whether "children of such tender years could be considered responsible agents, capable of making a decision in such a matter; or that vivisectors themselves had a legal right to accept the consent of these ignorant infants as warrant for inflicting this outrageous experiment."[16] In the scarlet fever case, as in the MacDonald whooping cough study, the children were volunteers in the sense that they had been volunteered by an adult, not because their preferences had been consulted. (The idea of a 3-year-old volunteering to be inoculated with a contagious disease strains even the most fevered imagination.)

For many investigators, obtaining parental consent or confining the research to their own children was not practical. Physicians who cared for children in orphanages, for example, faced questions about whether permission to study such children was necessary and who was authorized to give permission. When medical experiments involving orphans produced unambiguous benefits, no one expressed dissent; studies in which children experienced discomfort and risk raised troubling questions. Reports of experiments on orphaned children generated considerable public concern.

One of the few attacks on human experimentation not linked to antivivisection involved research in a New York City orphan asylum. In 1921 Konrad Bercovici, a New York journalist, published a stinging condemnation of medical experimenters who were using "orphans as guinea pigs" at the Home for Hebrew Infants. In order to study the development of scurvy, a common problem at orphanages, pediatrician Alfred F. Hess and his colleagues Mildred Fish and Lester Unger withheld orange juice from infants at the home until the babies developed the small hemorrhages characteristic of the disease. In addition to their efforts to create a diagnostic test for scurvy using subcutaneous punctures into the abdominal wall, Hess and Fish attempted to determine whether children could develop the disease again. They placed the infants on the scurvy regimen a second time and waited until symptoms developed. The doctors developed similar approaches for the study of rickets.[17]

The use of these orphans in nontherapeutic studies and the fact that the infants who developed scurvy often did not recover fully from the disease made such experimentation unacceptable to Bercovici. Praising "men of science" who sacrificed their own bodies in the search for knowledge, he declared, "But no devotion to science, no thought of the greater good to the greatest number, can for an instant justify the experimenting on helpless infants, children pathetically abandoned by fate and intrusted to the community for their safeguarding."[18]

Bercovici's explicit rejection of "anti-vivisection fanatics and the various freaks and cranks" hostile to medical progress may explain why his critique received a thoughtful hearing in the medical community. Even though the editors of *American Medicine* exonerated Hess and his colleagues of misconduct, they took Bercovici's protests seriously. Because the children's diets were carefully controlled, the journal's editors observed, the studies entailed little risk for the children, and the editors found them unobjectionable. They explained that the lack of an appropriate animal model and the fact that adults could not participate made research on children a necessity. In addition to the scientific utility of information about the dietary needs of infants, the research enabled the orphans to "make a large return to the community for the care devoted to them."[19] Although seldom expressed explicitly, the position that orphans could repay their debt to society through service as research subjects was held by many investigators and their defenders. So long as the risks were small or minimal, few physicians challenged the use of orphans and hospitalized children in medical research.

One of the problems, however, was defining acceptable levels of risk. Like Bercovici, antivivisectionists disputed physicians' descriptions of minimal risk. Citing medical articles that described the potential risks and dangers of lumbar puncture, antivivisectionists complained that performing such procedures for research purposes (rather than to diagnose an illness) on hospitalized children deserved condemnation from rather than publication by the medical profession. Instead, the leading medical journals disseminated the findings of investigators like M. Hines Roberts, who obtained spinal fluid from 423 sick and "normal" Negro infants at an Atlanta hospital "without regard to the character of labor or the condition of the child at birth."[20] Roberts's paper, which did not mention the consent of parents or guardians, described how "trauma produced by the needle at the site of puncture" was responsible for the blood in the spinal fluid in some of the infants.[21] In other words, newborn infants underwent a risky medical procedure for the purposes of scientific investigation.

Exposing children—orphans and others—to the dangers of untested vaccines and sera similarly alarmed antivivisectionists. "The wanton dosing of very young, healthy babies with filthy experimental messes of whose effect the vivisector himself is admittedly ignorant, is a gross violation of individual rights," responded one antivivisectionist to reports that a Baltimore physician had inoculated 107 infants with a vaccine of Flexner dysentery bacilli.[22] Vaccine-related complications and deaths, including the tragic deaths, in 1930 in Germany, of 76 children who had received contaminated BCG vaccine, confirmed antivivisectionist fears about scientific medicine. When American newspapers reported the development of two different vaccines for polio in 1934, stories about vaccine-related deaths ratified their worst suspicions.[23]

During the 1930s, investigators frantically sought a safe and effective vaccine to prevent the crippling disease of polio. To be useful, a vaccine had to produce immunity without creating full-blown disease. The respected pathologist John A. Kolmer championed a live polio virus vaccine, arguing that live virus was necessary to create lasting immunity. After experiments on a very small number of monkeys, Kolmer tested his polio vaccine on himself, his two children, and 23 other children "all immunized at the request or with the written consent of their parents."[24] He then extended the vaccine trial to 300 other children.

Operating in another laboratory with funding from the Rockefeller Foundation and Jeremiah Milbank, Canadian physician Maurice Brodie developed a killed-virus polio vaccine. With the aid of William H. Park, director of the Bureau of Laboratories of the New York Board of Health, Brodie conducted trials of his vaccine on adults (himself and six volunteers from the bureau). Twelve children "volunteered by their parents" also received the vaccine before Brodie initiated a large-scale trial involving 1600 children in Kern County, California. By 1935, when the vaccine trials ended, nearly 20,000 children had received one of the two experimental vaccines.[25]

Nine deaths among the participants, reportedly deaths from polio, led Kolmer to withdraw his vaccine in September 1935. Laboratory tests by independent researchers indicated that the Kolmer vaccine (containing live polio virus) was in fact dangerous. Unfortunately, the Brodie vaccine also failed to produce the necessary immunity to the disease. These claims for a safe and effective polio vaccine were apparently worthless. Unlike the German physicians whose flawed testing of the Calmette tuberculosis vaccine had resulted in the deaths of more than seventy children in Lubeck, the American investigators were not sued for damages.[26] But, argues polio researcher John R. Paul, this precipitate testing of vaccines on large numbers of children impeded vaccine research for nearly two decades.[27]

Amid the panic over the failed polio vaccines, antivivisectionists attempted to mobilize public opinion against the use of orphans in the tests. With the support of the mainstream animal protection movement, which had remained distanced from antivivisectionists, the issue of using orphans in medical experiments reached the Roosevelt White House.[28] A letter-writing campaign organized by the National Anti-Vivisection Society in 1933 prompted Eleanor Roosevelt to seek an investigation of the claims that orphans were being used in experiments with the newly developed polio vaccines of Drs. Kolmer, Park and Brodie. Polio, of course, held special meaning for the Roosevelts. The President's birthday balls raised large sums of money to fight the disease that afflicted Franklin Roosevelt.[29]

After receiving a number of letters about the testing of polio vaccine on orphans, Eleanor Roosevelt requested the surgeon general's office to investigate the claims. In response to a request from the assistant surgeon general, Kolmer explained that his tests proceeded only with parental consent. In addition to his own two sons, he tested the vaccine on his secretary's children and 18 others, but only with the express consent of the parents.[30] Park and Brodie also denied that they used orphans in tests of their vaccine.

William H. Park explained that clinical trials of their vaccine began only after the doctors had established "with absolute certainty that it was harmless."[31] Park was able to deny that he experimented on orphans because he believed that prior testing on adults and volunteered children insured that the vaccine was no longer experimental. Once the vaccines were withdrawn from public use in 1935, however, the question of when a vaccine ceases to be experimental received little sustained attention.

The revival of antivivisectionist activity in the 1930s and the concern about public reaction to using orphans in medical tests prompted some members of the research community to monitor the popular and medical press. At the Rockefeller Institute, for example, investigators paid close attention to newspaper articles and professional publications that could be misunderstood or misused by antivivisectionist critics. In 1932 Dr. Hyman L. Kramer, a member of the Harvard Infantile Paralysis Commission, informed a reporter for the *New York Times* that a serum treatment for infantile paralysis being tested by Simon Flexner was not ready for use on human beings. "Before we can give it safely to children, we shall probably have to give a shot of it to ourselves," he noted. "The Pasteur age is over. There can be no more disastrous wholesale experiments like Pasteur's rabies treatments to children before the serum was wholly proved."[32] Dr. Kramer's remarks alarmed Flexner's colleague at the Rockefeller Institute, Francis Peyton Rous. As editor of the *Journal of Experimental Medicine*, published under the institute's auspices, Rous worked hard to avoid problems with antivivisectionists. Weeks spent combatting antivivisectionist efforts in the spring of 1932 convinced Rous that Kramer's remarks would be used by the opposition at upcoming hearings before the New York legislature on proposals to restrict animal experimentation in the state. As it turned out, Kramer had been misquoted in the newspaper. Rous continued his vigilance and his care about the wording of articles in the *Journal of Experimental Medicine*.[33] The journal's articles were attracting an extraordinary amount of attention. Although it published few clinical research papers, reports of human experimentation were carefully edited with an eye to avoiding antivivisectionist criticism. In 1934, for example, Rous requested that researcher Yale Kneeland omit the word *infant* from the title of his paper on vaccination against colds. The editor similarly advised H. Mooser and his colleagues to alter their text describing the use of "lice fed on man" inoculated with a typhus strain to "lice fed on human volunteers."

In 1941, when he received a manuscript describing the infection of an infant "volunteer" with herpes virus, Rous sent a strongly worded letter of rejection to the author. The infection of a 12-month-old infant with herpes virus, he informed William C. Black, "was an abuse of power, an infringement on the rights of the individual, and not excusable because the illness which followed had implications for science. The statement that the child was 'offered as a volunteer'—whatever that may mean—does not palliate the action."[34] Black subsequently published his manuscript in the *Journal of Pediatrics*, including a description of his 12-month-old infant "volunteer." Rous's letter illustrates how seriously he regarded Black's offense,[35] but these strategies were undertaken largely to limit problems with antivivisectionist critics in order to protect animal experimentation. Appeasing antivivisectionists was easier than resolving the difficult questions raised by using children in medical research.

Children received extraordinary attention from animal protectionists because, like animals, they were vulnerable to medical exploitation. Often lacking the ability to speak or to make their wishes understood, children, especially infants, needed protectors. Antivivisectionists also extended their protection to some adult research subjects. Using prisoners, soldiers, and even paid volunteers could be morally problematic in the eyes of antivivisectionists.

The chief problem antivivisectionists identified in research on prisoners was the potential for coercion. The conditions of imprisonment made responsible and informed decisions about participation in prison medical research unlikely. One early target for antivivisectionists was the pellagra study conducted on a Mississippi prison farm. In 1915, pellagra was a serious problem in Mississippi. Doctors differed about the cause of the disease, which could lead to dementia and death. When U.S. Public Health Service investigator Joseph Goldberger approached Governor Earl Brewer of Mississippi for permission to conduct an experiment that would induce pellagra in male prisoners, he explained that observations at orphanages and hospitals had suggested that pellagra resulted from poor nutrition rather than a bacterium. Placing healthy male prisoners on a pellagra diet (meat, meal, and molasses) for six months would provide a convincing demonstration of this theory. Goldberger assured the governor that a healthy diet would reverse the disease process. The governor guaranteed pardons for male prisoners who followed the pellagra diet for six months.[36]

By the standards of the day, Governor Brewer's promise of a pardon was generous. In 1912 and 1913 American investigators from the biological laboratory of the Philippine Bureau of Science had offered much less to inmates of Manila's Bilibid prison who participated in their research. Like the Spanish volunteers in Walter Reed's yellow fever experiments, Bilibid participants gave written permission for the study. Unlike the yellow fever subjects, the Filipino prisoners did not receive "financial inducements," and they participated without "promise of immunity to prison discipline, or commutation of sentence."[37] Why the prisoners agreed to take part in research studies remains obscure; they may have welcomed the diversion, they may have believed it would help both medical science and their individual case, or they may have been misled. Nonetheless, before feeding gelatin capsules containing pathogenic amebic organisms to prison inmates, American physicians Ernest L. Walker and Andrew W. Sellards informed subjects "in their native dialect" about the experiment and the possibility of their contracting dysentery, and obtained written permission from them.[38] When investigators Richard P. Strong and B. C. Crowell used Bilibid prisoners to determine whether beri-beri was an infectious disease or the result of dietetic factors, they offered prisoners cigarettes and cigars as a reward for their willingness to remain on a rice diet.[39]

In Mississippi the governor's promise of a pardon for those in the pellagra study produced a large pool of volunteers. Goldberger selected twelve men, convicted of crimes ranging from bigamy and embezzlement to manslaughter and murder, and placed them on a diet consisting mainly of biscuit, cornbread, pork, and syrup. After six months, physicians confirmed the diagnosis of pellagra in six of eleven prisoners (one prisoner's escape attempt made him ineligible to continue in the study). When prison officials released the men, they offered free medical care to the prisoners during their recovery period, but none took advantage of the offer. "They all went off like a lot of scared rabbits," Goldberger noted.[40] Even before the experiment concluded, Governor Brewer received complaints. As historian Jon Harkness has shown, most critics of the experiment were more concerned about the apparent leniency to convicted felons (who escaped their rightful punishment by merely participating in a dietary study) than about medical exploitation of vulnerable human subjects.[41]

For antivivisectionists, exploitation was the issue. Incarceration in a state or federal prison (especially for prisoners serving life sentences) made it difficult, if not impossible, for individuals to make independent decisions about participating in research. The coercive nature of the pellagra study angered Diana Belais, president of the New York Anti-Vivisection Society. "It is not a case where men offered themselves freely in a spirit of self-sacrifice for the good of medical science. The men were convicts," she noted, "doomed to spend many years of their lives within prison walls."[42] Members of the California Anti-Vivisection Society raised similar concerns when they challenged experiments in testicular transplantation involving prisoners at San Quentin Prison. In 1920 physician L. L. Stanley described the implantation of human testes from recently executed convicts into eleven male prisoners. In addition to the human implants, the doctor transplanted ram testicles into 23 prison inmates suffering from various complaints.[43] To antivivisectionists, the testicular transplants illustrated how prisoners, like children in orphanages, soldiers, and the patients in mental hospitals, "furnished ample material for scientific curiosity."[44]

The occasional proposal to turn over to experimenters criminals soon to be executed also dismayed antivivisectionists. In 1917 when a professor at the Michigan Agricultural College demanded that hundreds of prisoners "who owe a big debt to mankind and who would make splendid subjects for vivisection" be substituted for mice and other animals in research on contagious diseases, antivivisectionists mourned the professor's "ethical blindness."[45] Reports of a "world-wide movement" to establish laws whereby criminals about to be executed could offer themselves for scientific experiment similarly alarmed some antivivisectionist observers, who identified a "new aggressiveness of vivisection" and labeled it a product of the Great War and "jazz reasoning."[46] Proposals to use "crooks for vivisection" won limited medical support in England, France, Cuba, and Mexico. In France, for example, a surgeon pressed the Chamber of Deputies to give murderers the choice between "the guillotine and the operating table." In Cuba, physicians proposed to inject condemned criminals with cancer "germs," and in Mexico, a resolution passed by the second national congress on *tabardillo* (typhus) urged reform of the penal code to allow experimentation on convicted criminals.[47]

Some of the antivivisectionists' disapproval of using "criminal guinea pigs" and other human beings resulted from their continuing suspicion of scientific medicine. When two convicts (Mike Schmidt, serving a life sentence for rape, and Carl Erickson, under the same sentence for murder) received pardons for participating in one 1935 experiment, some antivivisectionists questioned the scientific reasoning rather than the moral implications of using convicts in research. The experiment involved challenging a newly developed tuberculosis serum with injections of active tuberculosis bacilli. "The fact that these two men didn't get tuberculosis would be no proof that it was the vaccine and not their natural immunity which protected them," Robert Logan argued. "The theory of 'germ carriers' is evidence enough that people can be full of so-called deadly germs and not contract the disease which they are supposed to produce."[48] In an ironic twist, Morris Fishbein, a prominent medical journalist and sharp critic of the antivivisection movement, expressed many similar reservations about the scientific aspects of the tuberculosis experiment.[49]

The moral arguments against using prisoners in medical research were also invoked against involving members of the armed forces in medical experiments. Requiring military personnel, under threat of court-martial, to undergo experimental procedures troubled antivivisectionists. Joining forces opposing compulsory typhoid vaccination in the United States Army, antivivisectionists challenged both the idea that healthy individuals could spread disease and the "medical tyranny" that compelled American soldiers—suspected typhoid carriers—to undergo a risky gall bladder surgery to "cure" their condition.

During World War I, when military physicians identified soldiers as chronic typhoid carriers, they recommended surgical removal of the gall bladder. Physicians hoped that removing the gall bladder would render a typhoid carrier safe to others. Unlike civilian physicians, who lacked the authority to compel typhoid carriers "to subject themselves to the dangers incidental to such treatment," army physicians could order men to undergo the procedure.[50] The infamous Mary Mallon, the first identified American typhoid carrier, consistently refused to submit to gall bladder surgery. Although she was imprisoned by health authorities, the surgery was not performed. With military subjects, Lt. Col. H. J. Nichols and his colleagues explained the procedure, and some of the soldiers reportedly "consented willingly to operation when the condition was explained." Other enlisted men initially refused the surgery, but after "it was made clear to them that during the war they were subject to court martial if they refused an operation that might fit them for duty," the men agreed to the surgery.[51] It is difficult not to credit antivivisectionist claims that the soldiers' consent was coerced.

For the most part, however, during the first forty years of this century military experimenters regarded voluntariness as an important feature of acceptable human experimentation. As in the case of Walter Reed's yellow fever studies, many published papers of military physicians highlighted the use of volunteers in research. Army regulations in fact stipulated that researchers confine their studies to "volunteers for experimental inoculation or such other investigations as may have the approval of the War Department."[52] Although they did not define or explain their use of the word volunteer, military physicians often celebrated the "genuine devotion to science and humanity" that motivated soldiers to volunteer for non-therapeutic studies.[53]

The question about coercion in military medical research is difficult to answer. Experimentation on military personnel has received little attention from historians. Limited evidence suggests that soldiers retained the right to refuse participation in experimental projects and indicates that some army physicians tried to alleviate the concerns of potential volunteers.[54] In 1904, when army physician Edward Vedder attempted to introduce an experimental vaccine against typhoid fever, some of the men who had initially volunteered to receive the oral vaccine of dead typhoid bacilli later asked to be excused from participation. After Vedder and another army physician swallowed an amount larger than the prescribed dose, in an apparent effort to demonstrate the safety of the vaccine, the hesitant soldiers agreed to the test.[55]

Other research reports from military physicians imply that forms of coercion were employed to achieve compliance. In his report, army surgeon Charles F. Keiffer did not explain the nature of the "considerable resolution" he applied to insure the compliance of a sergeant and several privates who were taking part in his experiments involving the explosion of "smokeless powders" in a closed, sealed room to determine the effect of the gases on human beings. He also discounted the men's complaints of "severe headaches."[56]

Similar problems with the cooperation of "volunteers" arose in an experimental study of dengue fever conducted under American auspices in the Philippines. In 1931, James S. Stephens and Joe H. St. John, majors in the Army Medical Corps, remarked on the difficulties they were encountering in pursuing their research. Only the "diligent personal efforts" of medical officers enabled them to acquire the necessary volunteers from the armed services. Securing native Filipinos required greater effort: "After some difficulty four of the rather primitive Ifugao boys, from the barrio at Camp John Hay near Baguio, agreed to volunteer" for experiments on mosquito transmission of the fever.[57] We do not know how physicians persuaded "rather primitive boys" to agree to be bitten by dengue-infected mosquitoes. The authors did not mention payment or other incentives for their subjects. Dengue, unlike yellow fever, was not life-threatening, although it could be extremely unpleasant. Army researchers may have considered the pressing of "volunteers" into service for dengue research an acceptable practice.

Using soldiers as research subjects continued to raise issues of risk and

voluntariness. One way for physicians to avoid the ethical problems posed
by using uncooperative or potentially uncooperative subjects was to confine their studies to themselves, their students and colleagues, and "professional subjects." Paying adults of sound mind to participate in medical
research was not only permissible but desirable. "Every year firemen lose
their lives in the flames, and policemen are murdered," insisted vivisection
reformer Albert Leffingwell. "The compensation they receive induces them
to incur risk that would not otherwise be assumed."[58] Published research
reports suggest that investigators did offer financial compensation to their
human subjects in a variety of settings.

The practice of paying subjects for participating in nontherapeutic experiments was established before the Civil War.[59] One of the best-known
nineteenth-century experiments involved payment to the research subject.
In the 1820s, army surgeon William Beaumont was unable to close a gun-
shot wound in the stomach of a French-Canadian trapper named Alexis
St. Martin. In order to take advantage of this unique opportunity to study
the human digestive process, Beaumont was "obliged to pay high wages to
induce [St. Martin] to return and submit to the necessary examinations and
experiments upon his stomach and its fluids."[60] The army surgeon paid the
often-reluctant St. Martin $150, plus food, clothing, and lodging, for one
year of "reasonable experiments." After Beaumont's death, St. Martin was
"Barnumized" by a medical practitioner, T. G. Bunting, who, for financial
gain, exhibited St. Martin and his gastric fistula in a number of cities in the
eastern United States and Canada.[61] Not all antebellum attempts to procure
subjects proceeded as smoothly; in the 1840s, sailors and dockworkers in
Boston, for example, angrily rebuffed dentist William T. G. Morton's offer of
$5 to allow him to remove a tooth under the influence of his new anesthetic,
ether.[62]

In the South, slaves, of course, received no money when they were the
subjects of experimentation. They were not asked for, nor did they give,
consent to a physician's request. Some doctors offered compensation to
slaveowners for the opportunity to try new therapies on their slaves. In his
autobiography, physician J. Marion Sims described how, between 1845 and
1849, he kept several black female slaves at his hospital to test his discovery
of a repair for vesico-vaginal fistula. The fistulas, allowing urine or feces to
leak through the vaginal opening, caused great discomfort and distress.
Sims had proposed the following arrangement with one slaveowner: "If you
will give me Anarcha and Betsey for experiment, I agree to perform no
experiment or operation on either of them to endanger their lives, and will

not charge a cent for keeping them, but you must pay their taxes and clothe them. I will keep them at my own expense."[63] In order to perfect his technique to repair the vesico-vaginal injury, Sims performed dozens of operations on the women—this in the days before anesthetics—and praised their "heroism and bravery." Since he seemed to be failing to effect a cure, and in light of the money he was spending "to support a half-dozen niggers," his brother-in-law urged him to end the experiments, but Sims continued. The addition of silver sutures made the thirtieth operation on Anarcha and subsequent operations on Lucy and Betsey a success.[64] Unlike Sims, who maintained his subjects only during his experiments, some physicians preferred to purchase slaves who were afflicted with the medical conditions they hoped to study.[65]

In the late nineteenth and early twentieth centuries, some physicians continued the practice of paying men and women to undergo nontherapeutic procedures or tests. When Chicago physician Emanuel Snydacker, for example, wanted to see the effect of a trachoma culture on a human being, he "induced, by the payment of a sum of money" a 68-year-old blind woman "to allow herself to be inoculated with the pure culture."[66] He did not specify how much money was needed to induce her cooperation. Sometimes compensations were sufficient actually to constitute employment opportunities. In 1908, when the Referee Board of Consulting Scientific Experts, appointed by President Theodore Roosevelt and headed by chemist Ira Remsen of the Johns Hopkins University, conducted safety tests on saccharin, a sugar substitute, they authorized monthly stipends of $25–30 to adult subjects for their participation.[67] Private companies also employed research subjects in the testing of food products. In 1911 the federal government sued the Coca-Cola Company, challenging the claim that its beverage was the "ideal brain tonic." To refute the government's case, the company commissioned a study of the effects of caffeine on human mental function which included payment to the participants.[68] Psychologist Harry Hollingworth selected sixteen subjects, ten men (one teacher and nine students) and six women (identified as "wives"), ranging in age from 19 to 39. The subjects, who signed a document stipulating their agreement to abide by the nine research conditions, which included showing up for the experiment on time, received payment for their performance on a series of tests following ingestion of various doses of caffeine.[69]

Paying research subjects may have minimized problems for investigators but it did not eliminate them. In one case, the professional expertise of their paid research subjects thwarted the intent of two Boston physicians. In

1910 Edward Reynolds and Robert Lovett conducted a combined gyne-
cologic and orthopedic study of chronic backache. "A sense of propriety"
dictated that they limit their observations of hospital patients to views that
"could be made without undue exposure" of the patients. Therefore, to
supplement their observations with study of nude subjects, the physicians
engaged six female professional artist's models from the Boston Museum of
Fine Arts. They discovered, however, that the models' talent for assuming
"fixed unnatural positions," made them, ironically, less helpful for obtaining data about average women.[70]

In some cases, investigators may have had unrealistic expectations
about a paid subject's willingness to comply with a research project. When
Asa Chandler and Lee Rice attempted to study the etiology of dengue fever
in Galveston in the 1920s, they developed contractual agreements with
men and women newly arrived in the area. (It was important that subjects
not have prior experience with the fever, so the experimenters approached
passengers disembarking from evening trains.) For an undisclosed sum of
money, the subjects agreed to spend ten days in a screened room, to undergo blood and urine testing, to receive injections of blood from dengue
patients, and to permit infected mosquitoes to bite them. Given the strin-
gent conditions of the test, it is not surprising that some subjects "deserted
their contracts."[71]

Some people possessed unusual features that made them especially attractive as research subjects. One 31-year-old man's "unique ability to deliv-
er his stomach contents at will" (and his willingness to do it) encouraged
investigators to study him.[72] Men, women, and children with gastric fistulas continued to be of great interest to researchers studying the mechanisms
of hunger and digestion.[73] At the University of Chicago, physiologist Anton
Julius Carlson was "fortunate in having in his service" Fred Vlcek, a 27-year-
old Bohemian immigrant with a permanent gastric fistula "large enough to
permit direct inspection of the interior of the stomach, and the introduction of balloons, rubber tubes, and small electric lights for various investigations."[74] The interests of physiology, Carlson explained in 1912, demanded
that he secure the services of this "second Alexis St. Martin."[75] He guaranteed Fred Vlcek's participation by a monthly stipend.

Vlcek's experience at the hands of Carlson and his colleagues does not
bear out historian Ronald Numbers's suggestion that "researchers may have
grown more callous as the novelty of fistular experimentation wore off."[76]
Unlike the Continental physiologists conducting studies on patients with
fistulas, Carlson frequently expressed concern for Vlcek's well-being. The

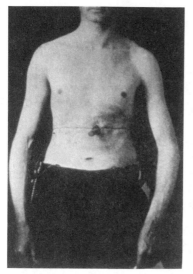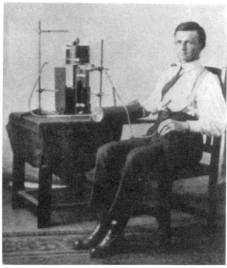

A. J. Carlson's professional subject, Fred Vlcek, with feeding tube in his permanent gastric fistula (*left*), and seated with laboratory apparatus (*right*). From A. J. Carlson, *The Control of Hunger in Health and Disease* (Chicago, 1916).

physiologist insisted on several occasions that such experiments as the introduction of local anesthetics "were compatible with *absolute safety* to Mr. V."[77] When studying the hunger contractions of the empty human stomach during prolonged starvation, Carlson explained that Vlcek could not be used in experiments involving lengthy periods of starvation because of the discomfort he suffered from hunger contractions: "Prolonged starvation is therefore so uncomfortable to Mr. V. that I did not feel justified to subject him to it, even though he expressed his willingness."[78] Rather than employ Vlcek, Carlson and a young assistant each undertook a five-day fast to determine the effect of starvation.

Self-experimentation and a good relationship with his research subject may have protected Carlson from the difficulties and adverse publicity encountered by a fellow investigator into the effects of starvation. A subject of nutrition researcher Francis G. Benedict, a young Italian lawyer named Agostino Levansin, complained bitterly to the press about the cruel treatment he allegedly received during a sixty-day fast in a respiration calorimeter, a room-size device for measuring heat loss.[79] Carlson did not wholly escape censure. Conceding that the physiologist "perhaps" obtained consent from his adult participants, antivivisectionists still questioned his experimental use of infants, who swallowed balloons for the study of hunger contractions.[80] Self-experimentation, however, did enable Carlson to undermine attacks that his research necessarily involved suffering. "Voluntary starvation is in no sense a heroic act," he insisted, "and citation of hunger experiments on animals in the interest of science as instances of cruelty to animals is without foundation."[81]

Ongoing research projects like Benedict's fasting studies required investigators to negotiate satisfactory terms with their human subjects. In 1939 when two research-minded Philadelphia physicians discovered a man with a longstanding gastric fistula, they were only able to persuade "Tom" to allow them to investigate his condition after nearly two years of coaxing. The man reluctantly agreed to become part of the study, the physicians explained, once he realized that the study of his fistula "might afford a means of improving his status and enhancing his security." The clinicians offered him a job as assistant and handy man in their laboratory. He proved amenable to most of the investigative procedures, especially after he became "emotionally dependent" on one of the two physicians.[82]

Paying human subjects for their participation in research and for their body fluids became routine in the 1920s and 1930s. "It is becoming common practice for probers into the unknown to make experiments of which persons with no thirst for knowledge are the victims," noted a report in the *Philadelphia Evening Bulletin*. Instead of making personal investigations, a scientist "hires one or more other persons to play with."[83] In addition to women who sold breast milk and the people who acted as "test subjects" for the standardization of toxins and antitoxins, physicians employed professional blood donors to supply fresh blood for transfusion.[84] Before World War II, blood was not routinely stored for clinical use, and cities across America maintained rosters of men (and a few women) who would supply blood at short notice for a fee. In Canada children as young as 8 and 10 also received payment for the serum they donated.[85] These paid donors occasionally performed additional roles. Some acted as research subjects and as "ghost" fathers in the 1930s, supplying sperm for artificial insemination to childless couples.[86] The dual role of professional donor and research subject sometimes created problems for investigators. After finding volunteer subjects from a Baltimore gymnasium "not altogether reliable," G. A. Talbert, a Johns Hopkins physiologist, paid medical student subjects to sit in a sweat-cabinet.[87] Some of Talbert's students were also serving as donors for blood transfusions at the hospital, a circumstance that produced unusual readings when they came to his laboratory shortly after giving blood.[88]

Medical students had long served as research subjects. Using this population sometimes required flexibility on the part of the investigator. When L. P. Herrington paid male medical students for their extended participation in some fifty-five to sixty hours of tests involving ionized air, he explained that his contracts with the men required them to appear twice a week for two to three months. He excused students, however, when "minor illness, overwork, or some special indulgence or recreation had occurred on the day or night previous to the experiment."[89] Female medical students similarly served as research subjects, because investigators experienced difficulty in enlisting enough other female volunteers.[90]

Worsening economic conditions in the late 1920s may have increased the availability of human subjects for research. The *New York Times* in December 1927 carried the advertisement of a healthy man willing to sell himself for medical tests. The 50-year-old man, who wished to remain anonymous, asked that researchers pay him $50 a week for the rest of his life.[91] During the Great Depression, employment bureaus sent jobless men to laboratories who paid for their services as subjects of research. The Department of Pathology at the University of Illinois College of Medicine, for example, used eighty unemployed men ages 20 to 76 in studies of the influence of weather on human beings. Sent by the state employment bureau, the men participated in studies of human response to various forms of stimuli.[92]

One agency of the federal government did not pay individuals to be research subjects but offered other forms of compensation. In 1932, the U.S. Public Health Service began a nontherapeutic study of untreated syphilis in black men, the now notorious Tuskegee Syphilis Study. In order to recruit and maintain subjects, investigators offered several incentives to Negro men in impoverished Macon County, Alabama.[93] Participants in the Tuskegee Syphilis Study, which continued until 1972, received "free hot meals on the days of examination, transportation to and from the hospital, and an opportunity to stop in town on the return trip to shop or visit with their friends on the streets."[94] Although the "Government doctors" withheld both information and treatment for syphilis from their subjects, they did dispense "free medicines" (pills and spring tonics for other conditions) to the men during their yearly visits to Tuskegee. The most significant inducement for compliance with the study, however, was the $50 in burial assistance given to the families who gave permission for post-mortem dissections. "Incentives for maximum cooperation of the patients must be kept in mind," nurse Eunice Rivers observed in 1953. "What appears to be a real incentive to an outsider's way of thinking may have little appeal for the patient. In our case, free hot meals meant more to the men than $50 worth of free medical examination."[95] In 1958 surviving subjects received a certificate recognizing their "voluntary service" and a dollar for every year they had participated in the study. Public outrage brought the study to a crashing halt in 1972. Surviving members of the experiment and their heirs sued the federal government for compensation for injury they had suffered. As part of the out-of-court settlement, surviving subjects eventually received $31,500 in partial compensation for their involuntary participation in the forty-year study.[96]

Paying men and women for their participation may have made investigators less sensitive to some of the ethical issues in human experimentation. Researchers, for example, seldom raised the possibility that the prospect of financial compensation made it impossible for some subjects to decline to participate. The money was intended to overcome the reluctance of potential subjects to take part in some experiments and to insure compliance with the research protocol. When subjects accepted payment, investigators may have believed that they had met their responsibilities to the subjects.

The social and cultural gulf between them did not encourage respect by investigators for their subjects. In the Tuskegee Syphilis Study, for example, attitudes of white investigators toward the black men who participated reflected assumptions about both race and class. Providing small incentives and the burial insurance encouraged investigators to adopt an instrumental attitude toward the subjects. Some of the social dimensions of the experimenter-subject relationship were recorded by gastroenterologist W. Osler Abbott in a remarkably descriptive account of the problems of using "professional guinea pigs" in the 1930s. In 1931 Abbott and T. Grier Miller, working at the University of Pennsylvania, developed a new technique for rapidly intubating the human intestine from mouth to rectum.[97] Although advised to try the new device on animals, the physicians apparently never performed the animal trials. After numerous self-experiments, they attempted to locate subjects in the hospital wards, and, failing, finally turned to healthy men and women who would agree to the procedure. Abbott and Miller approached a relief administrator in Philadelphia, hoping to gain cooperation in using unemployed men as subjects. She refused to send men to Abbott's laboratory after learning that the subjects would be required to swallow a flexible twelve-foot tube to which a rubber balloon was attached and inflated once inside the intestine.[98]

Frustrated at the employment bureau, Abbott asked the wives of his colleagues to distribute slips of paper instructing beggars to come to the hospital for a job paying $2 a day. He also used the bridge over the Schuylkill River as a "hunting ground" for potential participants, to no avail. At their secretary's suggestion the doctors called in their black janitor, Harry, eventually promising him "four bits" (50¢) for every healthy subject who appeared at the laboratory door at 8:30 a.m. in a sober and fasting state. Like the laboratory assistants who procured dogs and cats for experimentation, Harry arranged for a number of black men to take part in the intestinal studies, for which they received $2 a day.

Abbott's subjects created some problems. He complained that the men stole items from the dispensary. These subjects, he observed, also enjoyed a larger intake of corn liquor, pork chops, and chewing tobacco and led a less controlled existence than did the white rats in the medical school. On one occasion, Abbott was attempting to insert the tube into a man's duodenum using fluoroscopic guidance when he noticed a small piece of metal that he recognized as the tip of a .38 caliber revolver bullet. When confronted, the subject admitted that the previous night his jealous "sweetheart" had shot him, having seen him with another woman earlier in the evening. Such events, Abbott remarked, "led me to wish at times I could keep my animals in metabolism cages."[99]

More serious problems arose in the spring of 1935 when Abbott scheduled an exhibit on intestinal intubation for the American Medical Association, meeting in Atlantic City. After arranging for the men to be intubated before AMA members at a local hospital and then to appear at the convention, Abbott was stunned when the men refused to participate unless they received double pay. An impassioned eleventh-hour appeal to the third-year medical school class and the offer of the same pay received by the "striking blackamoors" enabled Abbott to continue the demonstration using student volunteers. He fired all the black subjects and refused to have anything more to do with them.

Several months later, however, Abbott reconsidered his position. "Those boys may have been short on morals but they were long in gut," and eventually he "went to Harry once again to throw out a feeler."[100] The "boys" were unable to continue the studies because they had "graduated from stealing inkwells to house furnishings." All but two had been convicted of burglary, and one subject was serving a ten-year sentence in the state penitentiary for a rape conviction.

An advertisement in a local newspaper brought a fresh group of potential subjects to Abbott's laboratory. Some of the men and women who answered the ad winced at the description of swallowing the tube, and many others apparently quailed at Abbott's insistence that they sign a statement prepared by the university attorney outlining every step of the experiment and stating that subjects recognized and accepted any risks associated with the procedure. (The document was more of an indemnification agreement to protect the university than a consent form.) Abbott ended up with a roster of subjects young and old, white and black, male and female, although he noted that his "clientele" eventually dwindled down to large, older women, the human counterpart, he said, of the "big, lazy, overweight bitch [from the animal house] that could be counted upon to lie and wag her tail while being worked over."[101] What Abbott's research subjects thought of the investigators and whether they actually understood the risks of tube-swallowing and of x-ray exposure is unknown. His equation of the lower-class men and women who participated in his tests with white rats and other laboratory animals certainly indicates that he did not consider them equal partners in the research process.

That investigators would treat human subjects like laboratory animals was precisely what antivivisectionists feared. Skeptical about the circumstances in which people agreed to act as professional guinea pigs, antivivisectionists complained that "hired persons are not always very clear in their minds as to what they are letting themselves in for."[102] When two Public Health Service researchers reported a study of pellagra, Nellie Williams, an officer of the American Anti-Vivisection Society, pointed out that their published report contained no information about the identity of the women who developed pellagra on the vitamin deficient diet, about where they lived, or about "how they happened to be chosen for the painful role of guinea pigs."[103]

The antivivisectionist focus on human experimental subjects encouraged some physicians to confront the ethical issues posed by research on human beings. Despite "unfortunate dealings" with antivivisectionists, whose statements he regarded as often "reckless" and "inaccurate," Harvard professor of medicine Richard Clarke Cabot publicly criticized cruel experiments on dogs and inappropriate research on patients.[104] "Experimentation upon a human being without his consent and without the expectation of benefit to him," Cabot observed, "is without any ethical justification." The fact that few physicians would dispute such statements did not mean that human vivisection seldom occurred. "The practice of making such experiments," claimed the New England Anti-Vivisection Society in 1926, "is common and is often condoned."[105] In order to address the moral problems of medical research, Cabot developed a code of conduct for hospital physicians. "Since hospitals furnish a unique opportunity for the prosecution of scientific research," he explained in 1931, hospital physicians needed to assume the responsibility of conducting research or to facilitate such research by other physicians.[106] In either case, physicians had the responsibility of insuring that no experiments were "done upon patients without their understanding and consent."[107]

Cabot's guide to medical ethics in the hospital did not address the issue of patient consent. Human experimentation continued to be left to the discretion of individual investigators. At least one case of nontherapeutic experimentation reached an appellate court before the end of World War II and the articulation of the Nuremberg Code. In 1941 John Bonner, a 15-year-old black junior high school student in the District of Columbia, underwent an experimental skin graft to help a severely burned cousin. Robert Moran, the cousin's plastic surgeon at the charity clinic of Episcopal Hospital, learned that Bonner had the same blood type as his burned patient and proceeded to take a skin graft from Bonner, without obtaining parental consent. When Bonner returned to the hospital to get "fixed up," he was subjected to a second operation. The physician, attempting a graft of living skin, formed a "tube of flesh" from Bonner to his cousin. Improper circulation in the tube created difficulties, and Bonner lost so much blood that he required several transfusions and had to spend nearly two months in the hospital.[108]

Bonner's mother, Margaret Moore, sued the physician for assault and battery. Even though she had not been asked for her consent, the trial court ruled in favor of the physician, noting that the 15-year-old's permission for the operation was sufficient. The District of Columbia Court of Appeals agreed that children could consent to medical therapy in exceptional cases, but these procedures did not involve a therapeutic benefit for John Bonner: "Here the operation was entirely for the benefit of another and involved sacrifice on the part of the [boy] . . . two months of schooling, in addition to serious pain and possible results affecting his future life. This immature colored boy was subjected several times to treatment involving anesthesia, blood letting, and the removal of skin from his body, with at least some permanent marks of disfigurement."[109] Eventually the hospital settled with Mrs. Bonner. Generally, in cases of nontherapeutic experimentation, physicians continued to be held responsible for adverse results. Written permission from the subject and evidence that the subject knew the risks before the experiment helped to protect a physician in court.

In the years between the first and second world wars, American antivivisectionists continued to monitor abuses of human subjects in medical research. Tests of new vaccines, drugs, and procedures on children, especially orphans, received the most attention, but these critics also raised questions about using prisoners, soldiers, and paid volunteers. Concern about charges that investigators employed human beings like laboratory rats prompted the research community to take steps to minimize the potential loss of public support. In addition to circumspection in the medical literature and the public press, the research community insisted that consent (or parental permission) and avoidance of risk were essential conditions of ethical human experimentation. The failure of some investigators to meet these conditions created problems, but defenders of medical research maintained that abuse was rare and pointed to their own willingness to serve as human guinea pigs as evidence of the good character of medical researchers.

Chapter Six

Heroes and Martyrs:
Human Experimentation in an Age
of Medical Progress

In the 1930s the American medical profession enjoyed unprecedented popular esteem. As historian John C. Burnham has observed, public opinion polls steadily confirmed that physicians were among the most highly respected professionals in America.[1] Advances in medical science—the discovery of insulin, sulfa drugs, and new treatments for pernicious anemia—helped inspire extraordinary confidence in the medical profession and in medical researchers. Despite pressure from antivivisectionists for restrictions on animal experimentation which continued to require physicians to make annual appeals to block legislation, medical investigators envisioned a bright future. Even the word *experiment*, once a word to avoid, had been rehabilitated by medicine's success. Although clinical experimentation was still a matter to "be approached with the utmost delicacy," as the dean of St. Louis University School of Medicine, Alphonse Schwitalla, observed in 1929, "a reasonable experimentation might well be regarded by the patient himself as a privilege that he would not, were the matter carefully explained, care to forego."[2]

How did experimentation on patients and other human beings move from dubiousness to privilege by the 1930s? Why did attacks against using orphans as guinea pigs fail to produce the legislative protections for human subjects in medical research that antivivisectionists desired? The dramatic success of medical science and the marginalization of the antivivisectionist movement in part explain public acceptance of human experimentation. Self-experimentation and the celebration of medical heroism and martyrdom also played an integral role in overcoming public anxieties about human experimentation.

Self-experimentation and research-related death and injury in medicine were not new, of course. What was new was professional investment in medical heroes and martyrs like Walter Reed (who survived the yellow fever studies) and Jesse Lazear (who did not). In the continuing controversy over animal and human vivisection, self-experimentation became a politically useful and emotionally satisfying asset for the defenders of animal and human experimentation. The ability to point to an investigator's willingness "to offer himself as a sacrifice" enabled them to take the moral high ground and to earn public support. Being the first to receive an experimental vaccine or drug offered a compelling illustration of the medical researcher's commitment to furthering medical knowledge and improving patient care. In the controversy with animal protectionists, self-experimentation undermined accusations of research exploitation and demonstrated the nobility of investigators.[3]

Clinical research was well established by the 1920s and 1930s, and the clinical investigator became an integral part of academic medicine.[4] With the creation of research units in hospitals, to conduct studies on patients, and the opening of new research hospitals, clinical investigators argued, patients actually received *better* care than patients in a hospital where research was not a priority.[5] At the same time, clinical investigators offered reassurance to the public about the limits of scientific experimentation on patients. When the University of Chicago opened its hospital in 1927, Rufus Cole, director of the Hospital of the Rockefeller Institute for Medical Research, noted how public attitudes toward hospitals had changed. "With the development and growth of modern scientific medicine and with the general recognition of the great blessings which it has bestowed, the dread of entering the hospitals and the reluctance to send our friends into them have largely disappeared." The rich and the poor, Cole declared, rushed to fill the available hospital beds, because they had learned that the best medical care was available in institutions where patients were studied scientifically. "This does not mean that patients must be the subjects for experiment—far from it," he hastened to explain. Experiments on animals insured that rash experiments on patients could be avoided. "It is only in hospitals directed by the ignorant and by charlatans that unusual and untested remedies are employed."[6] Clinical investigators and hospital administrators conceded that some public apprehension about research on patients continued. In 1946, nineteen years after the opening of the University of Chicago Hospital, Emmet Bay acknowledged that the hospital had developed, "to a certain extent," a reputation for using patients as guinea pigs. One advantage of this reputation, he claimed, was "the self selection of patients who represent more cooperative teaching and investigative material."[7]

Bay's observation points to a dimension of human experimentation that receives little attention. Some Americans apparently welcomed the opportunity to risk their lives for medical science and clamored for the opportunity to take part in the demonstration of a novel procedure or new drug. Responsible physicians may have had to fend off individuals hungry for attention or desperate for relief. In 1934, for example, when University of California researcher Robert E. Cornish announced a series of experiments to restore recently killed dogs to life, a number of Americans volunteered to take part in his revivification research. Attempting a further test, he was refused permission to test his procedure on the bodies of newly executed criminals. When this was widely reported in the popular press, Cornish received thousands of letters from men and women willing to undergo his experiments.[8] His volunteers included criminals sentenced to death, people in desperate need of money, and such pathetic individuals as a middle-aged Kansas woman, who wrote "I will submit myself for the experiment in any manner you say. I have always been in perfect health but—I am 46, so you see I haven't much to lose. It is immaterial whether I return or not."[9] Many physicians dismissed Cornish's experiments as quackery, but respected physicians also received offers from people willing or desperate for experimentation. During the 1940s and 1950s, the well-known infertility specialist John L. Rock received many letters from infertile women, begging the doctor "to use their bodies in experiments" in order that they might have a child.[10]

Of course, other Americans required assurance that experiments would not be lightly undertaken. Again, self-experimentation helped the researcher's cause. In the 1920s and 1930s the heroes and martyrs of scientific medicine became an important focus for the American medical profession. Few professionals, as historian George Weisz has observed, have been as devoted to celebrating their distinguished predecessors as have physicians. The collective process by which certain physicians (and not others) achieved prominence can tell us much about the self-perception and concerns of practitioners in a given era.[11] In the 1920s and 1930s the investment in heroes and martyrs amplified the authority of scientific medicine and illustrated the altruism of the medical profession. Defenders of medical research invoked the spectacle of scientific martyrdom to undermine accusations that investigators exploited human beings.

One explanation for the interest in the heroes and martyrs of medicine was the perception that the number of research-related injuries and deaths had climbed in the early twentieth century. As the number of laboratory workers multiplied and work with deadly diseases expanded, the risk of research-related injury and death increased. The growing sophistication of the bacteriological community meant that researchers were better able to identify disease outbreaks and deaths as resulting from their laboratory protocols. "Formerly cadaveric blood poisoning was almost the only recognized peril of the pathologist," observed the *Journal of the American Medical Association* in 1907, "others being incurred unknowingly, if at all."[12] The cultivation and handling of virulent microorganisms increased the likelihood of infection, either deliberately incurred through experimentation or accidentally acquired. In either case, physicians who developed disease or injuries in the laboratory were accorded the status of heroes or martyrs. In the 1920s the *Journal of the American Medical Association* even indexed research-related deaths under the entries "Heroes" and "Martyrs." In the *New York Times* index, research-related deaths could be located under the rubric: "Science, Martyrs To." Medical editors also classified deaths unrelated to scientific research but in the line of duty as a species of professional martyrdom: in 1929, a North Dakota physician who froze to death in a blizzard while making a house call to a patient was identified in the *JAMA* index as a martyr.[13]

In the first half of the twentieth century, two areas of medical research and practice produced the greatest concentration of heroes and martyrs, the use of the x-ray machine and bacteriological studies. By the 1920s it was clear that exposure to x-rays had harmed many of the people who had pioneered use of the machines. In these early decades, exposure times were considerably longer, and little shielding was employed to protect x-ray workers and their patients or subjects. Medical journals reported the sterility of x-ray workers, as well as the names of those injured and dead from radiation exposure. When G. C. W. Williams, a British radiologist, developed dermatitis from his work, he was fortunate to receive an allowance of $600 a year from the Carnegie Hero Fund while he underwent eight operations, including the amputation of his right hand and loss of two fingers on his left. A large number of European x-ray workers and many pioneering American radiologists received injuries.[14] One early pioneer of the x-ray and professor of radiology at the Johns Hopkins University, Frederick Henry Baetjer, for example, damaged both his hands and his eyes as a result of his exposure. He underwent several operations before he succumbed, "a martyr to research," in 1933.[15] Walter B. Cannon, who in 1896 had introduced the use of radio-opaque substances for the x-ray examination of the digestive process, died in 1945 from a rare malignant disease associated with his early x-ray research on digestion.[16]

Research on infectious disease similarly produced a large concentration of heroes and martyrs. U.S. Public Health Service investigator Howard Ricketts acquired typhus while investigating the disease in Mexico City in 1910 and died the same year. By 1928 research on Rocky Mountain spotted fever had cost the lives of four research workers: Thomas B. McClintic in 1912, William Gittinger and George Cowan in 1922, and Arthur LeRoy Kerlee in 1928.[17] Research-related deaths from typhus, tularemia, and polio were reported in both the medical literature and the popular press in the 1930s.

By 1941, seventeen "health soldiers" from the Public Health Service had died from infections contracted in the line of duty.[18] One female "martyr to science" was Anna Pabst, a bacteriologist at the Public Health Service.[19] Pabst died on Christmas Day in 1936 from meningitis, which she contracted "when a squirming animal into which she was injecting the meningitis culture caused misdirection of the serum into her eye."[20] Mishaps with laboratory animals contributed to the deaths of several investigators. Some of them continued in death to contribute to science: when a laboratory monkey bit an investigator at the Rockefeller Institute in 1934, researchers Albert Sabin and A. M. Wright performed an autopsy on their dead colleague.[21]

Those who survived their bouts with laboratory-acquired infections earned praise for their heroism. In the 1930s investigators at the Hooper Foundation for Medical Research at the University of California in San Francisco and at the Public Health Service laboratories in Bethesda developed the avian disease psittacosis several times in the course of laboratory experiments and survived.[22] Psittacosis was reportedly so contagious that the director of the Hooper Foundation would only permit himself and one assistant to perform the research work with birds "even though the assistants flirt with death-dealing germs dozens of times daily in their ordinary work."[23] Some researchers experienced multiple research-related illnesses. Edward Francis, a research worker at the National Institute of Health, developed tularemia in 1913, undulant fever in 1928, and parrot fever in 1930.[24]

The frequency of disease outbreaks associated with the study of brucella bacteria prompted Karl Meyer, director of the Hooper Foundation, to conduct a survey of American laboratories in which the microorganism was studied. In 1941 he reported seventy-four clinically, serologically, and bacteriologically proven brucella infections that could be traced to routine work or research with the bacteria. Forty-four of the seventy-four cases involved bacteriologists who handled the cultures or performed post-mortem dissections on infected animals. Animal caretakers, janitors, and technicians also developed the infection. Nearly half of those infected did not require hospitalization, but an equal number experienced "stormy prolonged illness."[25] Hospital stays and long recovery periods created financial hardships for those workers who were unable to obtain relief from worker compensation laws.

Research on yellow fever exacted a special toll on medical investigators. In the first decade of the twentieth century, efforts in Havana to study and prevent the disease caused four deaths. In addition to the death of Jesse Lazear, a member of the Reed expedition, three volunteers—the nurse Clara Maass and two Spanish men—died during trials of a yellow fever vaccine conducted by Juan Guiteras and William C. Gorgas.[26] Yellow fever research in the 1920s was also "paid for with precious lives."[27] In 1927 British professor Adrian Stokes, who demonstrated that yellow fever could be effectively transmitted to rhesus monkeys, succumbed to yellow fever while investigating the disease with the Rockefeller Commission in West Africa. "His death," noted the *Journal of the American Medical Association*, "adds one more name to the list of medical martyrs of science, who, like soldiers on the battlefield, have fallen in the performance of their work, and cuts short a brilliant career."[28] Less than six months later, in 1928, Rockefeller researcher Hideyo Noguchi, infamous in antivivisectionist circles for his syphilis studies, died in West Africa from yellow fever. Noguchi's death, reported on the front page of the *New York Times*, produced an outpouring of grief at the "tremendous blow to science." Nine days after Noguchi's death, newspapers reported that William Alexander Young, director of the Medical Research Institution of the Gold Coast and Noguchi's colleague in Accra, had also died a martyr to yellow fever.[29] Professional recognition of the occupational risks encountered by yellow fever researchers prompted two investigators to compile a list of cases of yellow fever contracted in experimental laboratories. Their list in 1931 included twenty-nine cases of research-related yellow fever, five of which resulted in death.[30]

The deaths of Noguchi, Stokes, and Young from yellow fever coincided with renewed efforts to commemorate the work of Walter Reed and the other yellow fever pioneers. Reed had never lacked admirers; after his death in 1902, friends and admirers solicited contributions for a memorial to him.

In the 1920s the movement to honor Reed and the surviving members of the yellow fever commission intensified, aided by the publication of medical journalist Paul de Kruif's *Microbe Hunters* in 1926.

Like Sinclair Lewis's popular novel *Arrowsmith* (published in 1925 and written with the help of Paul de Kruif), *Microbe Hunters* emphasized the heroic efforts of medical scientists, "who blazed a path through the darkness of ignorance, who experimented and failed—and tried again."[31] De Kruif's chapter on Walter Reed dramatically recounted the courageous medical soldiers, who first risked the "stabs of silver-striped she-mosquitoes" infected with yellow fever. In bold strokes, de Kruif painted Lazear's death and Carroll's near escape, the heroism of the American soldiers, who, he wrote, volunteered for the experiment "for the cause of humanity and in the interest of science," as well as the "ignorant [Spanish] immigrants— hardly more intelligent than animals," who received payment for their participation.[32]

The popular account of Walter Reed's experiments created considerable interest in the surviving members of the experiments. De Kruif's portrayal of the plight of Private John Kissinger, whose bout with experiment-induced yellow fever left him unable to support himself, prompted an investigation by several members of the American Association for Medical Progress, a lay organization incorporated in 1923 to defend animal experimentation. After a visit to the Kissinger home in 1926, a citizen committee, which included Harry Emerson Fosdick, William H. Welch, and a representative of the *New York Times*, was formed to raise money to aid the soldier and his wife. Kissinger had apparently been unable to work since his recovery from yellow fever and his return to the United States. His wife was compelled to take in washing to supplement the pension ($100 a year, granted in 1911) he received from the federal government. Newspapers and magazines publicized the "story of the soldier who gave himself to science" and helped the American Association for Medical Progress to raise $6,000 in order to buy a "dream home" for the "yellow fever martyr."[33]

Why did an organization devoted to the protection of animal experimentation raise funds for a "human guinea pig"? The surgeon William Williams Keen, who chaired the medical advisory board of the association, had long been interested in the potential of the Reed experiments to challenge antivivisectionist claims about the selfishness of medical investigators. In 1908 Keen had sought confirmation about the doctor volunteers from Reed's first biographer, Howard A. Kelly, who informed him that only Carroll had actually volunteered for the work.[34] Kelly maintained that Lazear's infection was accidental, although it could still be classified as a research-related death. Keen was able to use Kelly's biography to undermine the assertion that experimental work necessarily brutalized researchers. Walter Reed's letters to his wife, several of which Kelly published, expressed his concern for the safety and welfare of the men who had volunteered for the experiment. "The antivivisectionists have never dared to attack these experiments upon man," Keen observed in 1914. "If they had dared to do so, public opinion would have made short work of them."[35] Together with other members of the American Association of Medical Progress, the surgeon hoped that the "sentimental and historical appeals" for aid to the Kissinger family would garner favorable publicity for animal experimentation and would interest others in the cause.[36] To this end, the association attempted to locate other surviving volunteers of the Reed expedition and pressed for recognition of their service to the nation.

Participants in the yellow fever experiments went from relative obscurity to public celebrity in a short time. In 1928, for example, the city of Grand Rapids dedicated a bridge to the memory of William H. Dean, who was bitten by an infected mosquito in 1900. (Dean's infection apparently occurred without military authorization; he developed yellow fever nonetheless, but his name did not appear in early publications.)[37] Several local and state medical societies honored surviving volunteers in their home states. Although a 1928 proposal to create a special section in Arlington National Cemetery for the burial of soldiers who took part in the yellow fever studies did not receive congressional approval, the following year Congress did officially recognize the twenty-two members of the armed services who had participated in the studies and ordered that their names appear on the "roll of honor" published annually in the Army Register.[38] In addition to receiving gold medals, fifteen surviving volunteers were awarded pensions of $125 a year from the federal government.[39]

In the 1930s the yellow fever experiments became the subject of a Broadway play and a successful Hollywood film. The playwright Sidney Howard, who also wrote the screenplay for the film *Arrowsmith* in 1931, based his play *Yellow Jack* on Paul de Kruif's chapter on the Reed expedition. The play, which opened on Broadway in 1934, received considerable praise. "Graphic scenes of emotion, humor, laboratory ritual unroll new understanding of how old and new schools clash, how doctors and plain men sacrifice lives for other lives, what spiritual force it takes to ask such sacrifices," observed one New York critic.[40] At least one of the yellow fever survivors enjoyed seeing himself portrayed on Broadway. Sidney Howard had interviewed John Moran, one of the surviving soldier-participants of the studies, in 1932, during a visit to Cuba to see the actual site of Camp Lazear. In 1934 the producers invited Moran to attend a performance of *Yellow Jack*, where he met the young actor, Jimmy Stewart, who portrayed his character on stage. Stewart's thick Irish brogue apparently irritated Moran, but he enjoyed the performance anyway. Although *Yellow Jack* ran for only seventy-nine performances in 1934, a film based on the play was released in 1938 by Metro-Goldwyn-Mayer and received positive reviews.[41] The film, even more than the play, focused attention on the heroism of the ordinary men like Moran and Kissinger who had volunteered for the yellow fever studies. Ironically, authorities in Cuba apparently banned *Yellow Jack* because the producers had failed to credit the Cuban physician Carlos Finlay for his early, but unproven, theory that the disease was transmitted by mosquitoes.[42]

John Moran and John Kissinger, who had (initially) insisted that they receive no payment for their participation in the yellow fever studies, achieved minor celebrity. They made several public appearances, at times together. In 1937 the popular radio personality Lowell Thomas invited Moran to be on his program to give a brief history of his role in the yellow fever studies. Moran, who was coached for more than an hour by a shadowwriter, received more than three hundred letters after his talk.[43] Honored by the University of Virginia Department of Medicine in 1940, Moran, together with Kissinger, also attended the dedication of the Jesse W. Lazear Laboratory Building at Washington and Jefferson College, where the college drama club presented *Yellow Jack* in honor of the occasion.[44]

Kissinger was also invited, along with Walter Reed's daughter, to the public unveiling of Dean Cornwell's painting "Conquerors of Yellow Fever." The third painting in the "Pioneers of American Medicine" series depicting great moments in medical history (the first two were "Beaumont and St. Martin" and "Osler at Old Blockley"), Cornwell's painting was officially unveiled at the 1941 annual meeting of the American Medical Association.[45] Articles in the medical and popular press emphasized the efforts to insure the historical accuracy of the painting, which included portraits of fifteen men.[46] In addition to Reed, Lazear, Carroll, and several army officers, Cornwell painted four American experimental subjects (Moran, Kissinger, Warren Jernegan, and Dr. Robert Cooke) and one nameless Spanish immigrant (representing the four Spanish men who also volunteered).

The film *Yellow Jack* was one of a spate of popular motion pictures in the 1930s that celebrated the heroism and nobility of the medical profession. As

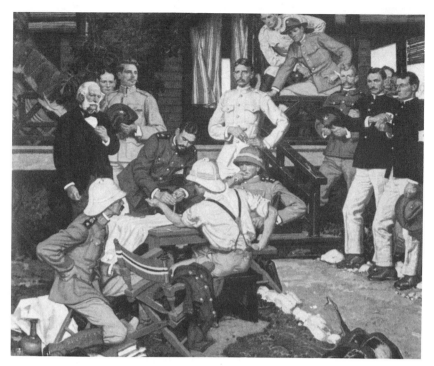

"Conquerors of Yellow Fever," a painting by Dean Cornwell. Published in *Hygeia*, 1941; reprinted by permission of Wyeth-Ayerst Laboratories.

historian Richard H. Shryock observed, the popularity of films like *Men in White, Women in White, The White Parade*, and *The White Angel* made it seem "as though anything 'in white' was good for box-office returns."[47] Defenders of medical research sought to capitalize on these film images in their battle against restrictions on animal experimentation. In 1938, for example, leaders of several California medical schools called on the president of Metro-Goldwyn-Mayer, asking that some of the prominent male actors who had "gained worldwide recognition" in their roles as doctors in these films aid the fight to insure the sale of pound animals to medical institutions.[48] Louis Mayer failed to provide Clark Gable (the star of *Men in White*) or Robert Montgomery (who played John Moran in *Yellow Jack*), but MGM produced two motion picture shorts extolling the scientific exploits of Louis Pasteur, and Banting and Best, the discoverers of insulin. *Man's Greatest Friend*, an eleven-minute film depicting Pasteur's discovery of a vaccine for rabies, included portraits of two yellow fever martyrs, the "heroic humans of science," Hideyo Noguchi and Jesse Lazear.[49]

The revival of antivivisectionist activities during the 1930s made the yellow fever experiments and the heroism of the physicians and soldiers an attractive topic in the publicity of the defenders of medical research. William Keen challenged the antivivisectionists with the "heroic self-sacrificing death of Noguchi and his assistant. Who is the A-V," Keen bitterly observed, "who has even inconvenienced him- or herself in the service of humanity much less offered up his or her life in ferreting out the nature of a remedy for the African form of yellow fever or *any* other disease?"[50] The American Association for Medical Progress issued a special pamphlet on vivisection and yellow fever that similarly emphasized the human and animal sacrifices that made control of yellow fever possible.[51]

Medical critics of the antivivisection movement explicitly invoked the heroism of medical investigators like Lazear, Carroll, and Noguchi in their efforts to defend unrestricted animal experimentation. Unlike antivivisectionists, who threatened to prevent medical progress, wrote physiologist Virgil Moon, researchers "braved the unseen and mysterious dangers of disease with as high courage as man can summon. Neither reward nor fame awaited them; no acclaim of shouting multitudes greeted their success. When, as often happened, they succumbed to the disease they sought to conquer, no marble shaft marked their resting place and no bronze tablet recorded the story of their sacrifice."[52] Articles in *Hygeia*, a journal issued by the American Medical Association for a lay audience, highlighted the heroism of microbe hunters, "who daily cheat death while delving into the cause and cure of mysterious ailments like parrot fever, tularemia, typhus and rabbit fever." Pharmaceutical companies, which also had a stake in the antivivisection controversy, contributed to the effort. The Philadelphia-based Wyeth Company, for example, provided funding for the Pioneers of American Medicine series that included the "Conquerors of Yellow Fever."

Despite all this acclaim for scientists, antivivisectionists continued to regard the motives of medical researchers with suspicion. Some praised the heroic efforts of physicians who risked their own lives during self-experimentation: "Anti-vivisectionists," noted Agnes Chase, a frequent contributor to the antivivisectionist journal *The Starry Cross*, "have no quarrel with the true scientist whose deep interest and hope in medical discoveries lead him to carry out upon his own person the experiments he deems necessary to achieve success."[53] Chase commended Alabama physician A. W. Blair, for instance, who allowed himself to be bitten by a poisonous black widow spider. Ironically, Blair revealed that his experience of "excruciating pain" and a close escape from death made him reluctant to undertake future self-experiments.[54]

What antivivisectionists found troubling about self-experimentation was the tendency of researchers to make the leap from their own bodies to those of others. In 1934, when physician John Kolmer announced that he had developed a vaccine to immunize children against polio, he asserted that tests on himself and his secretary had established the safety of the vaccine. Given Kolmer's own observation that the majority of adults were immune to polio made antivivisectionist critics skeptical about the legitimacy of extending the vaccine to children.[55] They, like the investigators, realized the public relations value of reporting self-experiments. Americans were more willing to accept a vaccine that investigators had tested on their own bodies. For similar reasons, William H. Park, Kolmer's competitor in the race to develop a polio vaccine, revealed that he and two other city doctors, "one of them a woman," had administered their vaccine to themselves, "so that the public would not have any fear of the vaccine."[56]

Scrupulousness in discussing research on human subjects also helped assuage fears about research exploitation. Medical editors like Peyton Rous monitored discussions of human experimentation in the medical literature. Hospital administrators exercised care in presenting research to lay audiences. In 1946, for example, the staff of the Veterans Administration explained, "We don't like to use the word 'experiments' in the Veterans Administration; 'investigations' or 'observations,' . . . is the approved term for such a study in the VA hospitals."[57]

The American public welcomed the advances in medicine that had occurred by the 1930s. Many people seemed willing to bear the human costs of training young doctors and acquiring new knowledge. The problem, one observer noted, was, "If it is true that the progress of medicine has been over a mountain of corpses, one objects to its being one's own corpse. If it is also true that in medicine 'nothing risked, nothing gained,' one prefers to have the gain to humanity made at the expense of somebody else."[58] The apparent willingness of the medical profession to assume some of the responsibility for going first and the impressive record of medical heroism and martyrdom in the early decades of the twentieth century persuaded many Americans that human experimentation was not the horror that antivivisectionists claimed. Although experiments on orphans continued to be problematic, few Americans shared antivivisectionist concerns about the professional subjects, prisoners, soldiers, and the other adult populations who participated in research.

The antivivisectionist crusade against human vivisection exercised a curious influence on the conduct of medical research in the first four decades of the twentieth century. Fearful that accusations that medical researchers exploited research subjects would lead to restrictions on animal experimentation, the leading members of the research community considered but rejected the development of a formal code of ethics for human experimentation. They adopted several strategies to limit the damage caused by physicians who seemed to transgress. The human vivisection controversy prompted explicit discussions about the requirements for ethical human experimentation. Taking responsibility for the welfare of the subject, obtaining prior consent of the subject or guardian, and being willing to go first continued to be essential to professional definitions of appropriate human experimentation. By the 1930s, the public's confidence in medical research and admiration for the medical profession in general made the task of defending medical research much easier than it had been at the turn of the century.

Epilogue

In 1916 vivisection reformer Albert Leffingwell called for legislation to prevent human vivisection—federal and state laws that, with stiff penalties for infractions, would protect infants, children, and other vulnerable human beings from exploitation at the hands of experimenters. "No such law need interfere in the slightest degree with the rights of the true physician to aid his fellow-beings," Leffingwell insisted. "Nor can we doubt that the medical profession will finally favour a reform that will indicate the broad line of demarcation separating the unquestioned privilege from the unjustifiable abuse."[1]

In 1966, fifty years after Leffingwell's call for protective legislation, a Harvard medical professor published an exposé of abuses in clinical research in one of America's leading medical journals. Henry Beecher's essay in the *New England Journal of Medicine* precipitated a thoroughgoing reform of American medical research ethics that culminated in federal protections for the human subjects of biomedical and behavioral research.[2] Together with the revelation of research scandals like the hepatitis study involving retarded children at the Willowbrook School and the forty-year study of untreated syphilis involving four hundred African-American men, Beecher's report spurred Congress to pass the National Research Act. The act, signed into law by President Richard Nixon in 1974, established the National Commission for the Protection of Human Subjects in Biomedical and Behavioral Research. In 1978, the commission issued the landmark Belmont Report, which identified three cardinal principles for human experimentation: respect for persons; beneficence/nonmaleficence; and distributive justice.[3] Armed with these principles and a wealth of articles from medical ethicists, university and hospital institutional review boards began the task of approving or rejecting protocols involving human subjects.

As we have seen, much changed in American medical research during the 1920s and 1930s. During the 1940s, America's entry into World War II made experimentation less a privilege that middle- and upper-class patients would be willing to pay for than a patriotic responsibility for all Americans. Men, women, and children were pressed into service as research subjects as researchers joined the war effort. Established by President Franklin Delano Roosevelt in 1941, the Office of Scientific Research and Development coordinated medical research through the Committee for Medical Research (CMR). Charged with "mobilizing the medical and scientific personnel of the nation," the CMR, under the direction of pharmacologist A. Newton Richards, administered 450 contracts to universities and 150 to research institutes, hospitals, and other organizations. In order to solve pressing military medical problems, the CMR committed funds for nontherapeutic research involving orphans, the retarded, prisoners, and the mentally ill. As David J. Rothman has persuasively argued, moral qualms about using these populations in nontherapeutic studies faded in the harsh light of wartime necessity.[4]

The wartime investments in medical research produced impressive results. The development of penicillin, cortisone, gamma globulin, blood substitutes, and other drugs and techniques impressed both Congress and the American public. Funding for medical research rapidly expanded in the years after World War II, increasing the number of medical investigators and multiplying the number of experiments involving human subjects. In 1946 the National Institutes of Health received approximately $700,000 from the federal government. By 1955 the NIH appropriation exceeded $36 million; in 1970, NIH received nearly $1.5 billion from the federal government and administered over 11,000 grants.[5]

The unprecedented growth in medical research expenditures and the increasing use of human subjects did not initially generate much discussion about the ethics of human experimentation. The revelation of the Nazi atrocities, their nature and hideous extent, and the prosecution of the Nazi doctors encouraged the formulation of international standards for ethical human experimentation.[6] In 1946, the American Medical Association adopted the requirement of voluntary consent for experimentation, but researchers seemingly paid scant attention to this development.

For their part, American antivivisectionists continued to protest the use of animals in research, but they no longer criticized animal experimentation on the basis that it would lead to the exploitation of human subjects. References to human research subjects in antivivisectionist journals declined during the 1950s and 1960s as animal activists began to redefine the nature of the human-animal relationship. Rejecting the "humane" tradition which treated animals as objects of pity, newly formed animal welfare groups insisted that animals were entitled to consideration as beings with interests and emotions. In the 1970s, the emergence of the animal rights movement completed the transformation; "the gradual radicalization of the animal protection movement thus followed changing images of animals; from pitiable objects of charity, to innocent beings with interests of their own, and, finally, to autonomous individuals with a right to their own lives."[7] The new focus on animal rights made the abuse of human subjects less compelling for animal rights activists than it had been for turn-of-the-century antivivisectionists.

The year 1966 marked an important landmark in the history of both human and animal experimentation. Following a graphic exposé in *Life* magazine of the poor conditions at the puppy mills which supplied medical laboratories, Congress passed the Laboratory Animal Welfare Act.[8] This first federal legislation concerning the care of laboratory animals required registration of research facilities and licensing of dog dealers. Although it did not address research procedures in the laboratory, the act set minimum standards for food, water, and maintenance for some animal species. (The act has undergone considerable revision since 1966; major amendments occurred in 1970, 1976, and 1985.)

It was also in 1966 that Henry Beecher published his challenge to clinical researchers. In a carefully orchestrated article in the *New England Journal of Medicine*, the Harvard anesthesiologist described twenty-two research teams in which investigators "risked the health or life of their [human] subjects."[9] Beecher's report and the subsequent public outcry over a series of experiments involving the abuse of human beings hastened the establishment of federal protections for the human subjects of biomedical research.[10] Americans learned from the popular press of conditions at the Willowbrook School, where retarded children were experimentally infected with hepatitis, and of cancer experiments at the Jewish Chronic Disease Hospital, where elderly patients were injected with live cancer cells. The revelation in 1972 that the U.S. Public Health Service had conducted a forty-year study of untreated syphilis in black males spurred the U.S. Department of Health, Education, and Welfare (now the Department of Health and Human Services) to release in 1973 the first set of proposed regulations concerning the protection of human research subjects.[11] The National Research Act, passed in 1974, mandated formal protections for human subjects, including written consent and institutional review boards, composed of both medical professional and lay persons, to evaluate proposals involving experiments on human beings. Since 1974, the guidelines have undergone some modification but the basic machinery of institutional review boards remains intact.

The advent of federal regulation has not resolved the ethical issues raised by human experimentation. Diseases—both old and new—and innovative technologies raise troubling questions about where to draw the line between appropriate human experimentation and unjustifiable abuse. A number of critics complain that the ideal of informed consent for participation in medical research is not attainable in practice. How, these observers ask, can a dying cancer patient make balanced judgments when invited to participate in a trial of an aggressive new therapy? Other critics have charged that the desire to protect vulnerable populations from experimental exploitation has helped create "therapeutic orphans." Exempting children from clinical drug trials, for instance, prevents physicians from prescribing potentially effective drugs in treating them. These difficult issues are unlikely to be easily resolved in the near future.

"There is no objection to human experimentation," observed Albert Leffingwell, "when there is no invasion of human rights."[12] The controversy over human vivisection in the first four decades of the twentieth century illustrates the process by which human rights are defined and redefined in light of cultural assumptions and professional allegiances. In the early twentieth century, American antivivisectionists warned about the transformation of the physician into the scientist at the bedside. In the last decade of the twentieth century, the bedside is considerably more crowded, but questions about human rights and what it means to be both human and humane continue to disturb the peace.

Appendix

A Bill for the Regulation of Scientific Experiments
upon Human Beings in the District of Columbia

The following bill (S. 3424) was introduced by Senator Jacob H. Gallinger to the Senate of the United States on 2 March 1900 (56th Cong., 1st sess.) and was referred to the Committee on the District of Columbia.

Be it enacted by the Senate and House of Representatives of the United States of America in Congress assembled, That no physician, surgeon, pathologist, student of medicine or of science, or any other person shall make or perform upon the body of any human being, in any hospital, asylum, retreat, or infirmary established for the treatment of the sick, or in any other place in the District of Columbia, any scientific experiment involving pain, distress, or risk to life and health, whether by administration of poisonous drugs for the purpose of ascertaining their toxicity, by inoculating the germs of disease, by grafting cancerous tumors into healthy tissues, or by performance of any surgical operation for any other object than the amelioration of the patient, except to the restrictions and regulations hereinafter prescribed. Any person performing, advising, or assisting in the performance of any such experiment upon any new-born babe, pregnant woman, lunatic, idiot, or patient, in any public or private hospital, in any infants' home, hospital, asylum, or private house, or upon any other person whatsoever, shall be deemed guilty of the crime of human vivisection, and upon conviction shall be liable to a fine of not less than one thousand dollars or imprisonment for not less than one year, or both. If any such experiment shall be followed within forty-eight hours by the death of the person thus operated upon, or if it shall appear that death was accelerated in any way by such experiment, the performance of any such experiment shall be deemed manslaughter or murder, as the circumstances of the case shall determine; and all persons taking part therein shall be liable to the penalties prescribed for such crime.

SEC. 2. That any physician or surgeon duly qualified to practice medicine in the District of Columbia, or any medical student, who shall perform any such scientific experiment, or who by his advice or presence shall in any way assist, aid, or abet the performance of any such experiment, shall, upon conviction, be forever disqualified from the practice of medicine in the District of Columbia. Any person engaged in any capacity in the service of the United States Government or in any of its departments who shall perform, or by his presence, suggestion, or advice, aid or abet the performance of any such experiment upon a human being, shall, upon conviction, in addition to other penalties herein provided, be forthwith dismissed from Government service and be forever disqualified therefor.

SEC. 3. That any description or account of any such experiment upon a human being, printed or published in any scientific or medical periodical or book, or in any reputable newspaper, shall be deemed evidence demanding immediate inquiry into all the circumstances of the alleged crime, and, if corroborated by further evidence, shall be accepted as testimony in regard to the offense.

SEC. 4. That an experiment performed upon a human being with a view to the advancement by new discovery of physiological or pathological knowledge shall, if it involves pain or distress, be permitted only under the following restrictions:

(a) The experiment must be performed only by a duly qualified physician or surgeon holding such special license from the Commissioners of the District of Columbia as in this Act mentioned; and

(b) The subject of such experiment must be not less than twenty years of age and in full and complete possession of all his or her reasoning faculties. No scientific experiment of any kind liable to cause pain or distress shall be permissible upon any new-born babe, infant, child, or youth; nor upon any woman during pregnancy nor within a year after her confinement, nor upon any aged, infirm, epileptic, insane, or feeble-minded person under any circumstances whatever.

(c) The physician or surgeon proposing to make any such experiment or series of experiments shall, at least one week in advance, apply to the Commissioners of the District of Columbia for license permitting such experiment or experiments to be performed. Such application shall fully state the objects and methods of the proposed experiments, and shall be accompanied with the written permission of the subject of the proposed experimentation, agreeing thereto, signed in presence of two witnesses and duly acknowledged before a public notary under seal.

(d) Upon receipt of such application, the Commissioners of the District of Columbia shall cause investigation to be made; and if it shall appear that the experiments involve no risk to human life; that the person offering himself or herself for experimentation is of requisite age, in full possession of all his or her reasoning faculties, and fully aware of the nature of the proposed experiment, and desires that it be made, then the Commissioners may issue a license authorizing such scientific experiment or series of experiments as desired; but

(e) No such experiment shall at any time be continued against the expressed will of the person experimented upon.

(f) The Commissioners of the District of Columbia shall require a report to be made to them of the methods employed and the results attained of each experiment or series of experiments thus made. Such report may not be made public until after six months from the beginning of the experimentation, in order to permit the investigator to present the results of his work in his own way. But in the event of any untoward circumstance attending any such experimentation the full details shall immediately be reported and printed.

SEC. 5. That nothing in this Act contained shall be construed to prohibit or interfere with any properly conducted method of medical treatment or surgical operation, whether experimental or otherwise, having for its demonstrable end and object the amelioration of suffering or recovery of the patient thus treated or operated upon.

SEC. 6. That nothing in this Act contained shall be construed to prohibit or interfere with any experiments whatsoever made by medical students, physicians, surgeons, physiologists, or pathologists upon one another.

Notes

1. This Bill has but one object, the protection of those who cannot protect themselves.

2. No reputable physician or surgeon is affected by it. It will not interfere in the slightest degree with any method of treatment designed for the benefit of the patient. Read carefully Section 5.

4. It does not even prevent scientific experiments upon human beings (when these are not dangerous to life), if the full and free consent of the subject shall be first obtained and attested by oath before a proper authority. But it forbids absolutely all experiments productive of pain or distress, or dangerous to life and health, upon

children of any age, or the inmates of asylums, hospitals, or public institutions; in short,—upon those who from weakness or ignorance cannot protect themselves, and whose helpless condition appeals to the common instinct of humanity everywhere.

5. The proof of necessity for restraining legislation in this matter may be had by sending ten cents in postage stamps for literature on human vivisection as practiced in America and Europe.

Address

SPECIAL COMMITTEE,
AMERICAN HUMANE ASSOCIATION,
Providence, R.I.

Notes

Abbreviations

APS   American Philosophical Society, library, Philadelphia

ASPCA   American Society for the Prevention of Cruelty to Animals, archives, New York

CPP   College of Physicians of Philadelphia, library

CPS   College of Physicians and Surgeons, Columbia University, Augustus C. Long Health Sciences Library

HMS   Harvard Medical School, Francis A. Countway Library

MHC   Michigan Historical Collections, Bentley Historical Library, University of Michigan, Ann Arbor

RUA   Rockefeller University Archives, North Tarrytown, New York

UCSF   University of California at San Francisco, library

UR   University of Rochester School of Medicine and Dentistry, Edward G. Miner Library

UVA   University of Virginia, Claude Moore Health Sciences Library, Charlottesville

Introduction

1. For an important exception, see Gert H. Brieger, "Human Experimentation: History," in *Encyclopedia of Bioethics*, ed. Warren T. Reich (New York: Free Press, 1978), pp. 684–92.

2. George J. Annas and Michael A. Grodin, eds., *The Nazi Doctors and the Nuremberg Code* (New York: Oxford University Press, 1992).

3. William Bynum, "Reflections on the History of Human Experimentation," in *The Use of Human Beings in Research: With Special Reference to Clinical Trials*, ed. Stuart F. Spicker, Ilai Alon, Andre de Vries, and H. T. Engelhardt, Jr. (Dordrecht, Netherlands: Kluwer Academic, 1988), pp. 29–46.

4. On the use of the word *vivisection*, see William W. Keen, *Animal Experimentation and Medical Progress* (Boston: Houghton Mifflin, 1914), p. vi.

5. Albert T. Leffingwell, *An Ethical Problem* (New York: C. P. Farrell, 1916), p. 290.

6. The film, *Island of Lost Souls*, based on Wells's 1896 novel was released by Paramount Productions in 1932; Sidney Howard, *Yellow Jack* (New York: Harcourt, Brace, 1933), p. 46.

7. James H. Jones, *Bad Blood: The Tuskegee Syphilis Experiment*, new and exp. ed. (first pub. 1981; New York: Free Press, 1993), p. 97.

8. Sinclair Lewis, *Arrowsmith* (1925; New York: New American Library, 1980), p. 360.

Chapter One

1. John Harley Warner, *The Therapeutic Perspective: Medical Practice, Knowledge, and Identity in America, 1820–1885* (Cambridge: Harvard University Press, 1986), p. 264.

2. William Osler, "The Evolution of the Idea of Experiment in Medicine," *Trans. Congr. Am. Phys. Surg.*, 1907, *7*, 7.

3. Ibid., p. 8.

4. Kenneth M. Ludmerer, *Learning to Heal: The Development of American Medical Education* (New York: Basic Books, 1985), p. 103.

5. William Rothstein, *American Physicians in the Nineteenth Century: From Sects to Science* (Baltimore: Johns Hopkins University Press, 1972; reprint 1992), pp. 261–81; and Patricia Peck Gossel, *The Emergence of American Bacteriology, 1875–1900* (Ph.D. diss., Johns Hopkins University, 1989), pp. 165–99.

6. Justina Hill, "Experimental Infection with Neisseria Gonorrhoeae," *Am. J. Syphilis*, 1943, *27*, 733–71; and Vikenty Veressayev, *The Memoirs of a Physician* (New York: Alfred A. Knopf, 1916).

7. Henry Heiman, "A Clinical and Bacteriological Study of the Gonococcus Neisser in the Male Urethra and in the Vulvovaginal Tract of Children," *J. Cut. Genito-Urinary Diseases*, 1895, *13*, 384–87; see also *Med. Rec.*, 1895, *47*, 769.

8. Lawrence K. Altman, *Who Goes First? The Story of Self-Experimentation in Medicine* (New York: Random House, 1987), pp. 23–26.

9. George M. Sternberg and Walter Reed, "Report on Immunity against Vaccination Conferred upon the Monkey by the Use of the Serum of the Vaccinated Calf and Monkey," *Trans. Assoc. Am. Physicians*, 1895, *10*, 57–69.

10. "Propositions in Regard to Animal Vaccination," *Med. Rec.*, 1874, *9*, 22.

11. W. K. Jaques, "Experiments and Observations in Scarlet Fever," *JAMA*, 1900, *34*, 1302.

12. Gerald B. Webb, "Studies in Tuberculosis," *Bull. Johns Hopkins Hosp.*, 1912, *23*, 233.

13. Warner, *Therapeutic Perspective*, p. 271.

14. George F. Shrady, "The Earlier Employment of Cocaine," *Med. Rec.*, 1884, *26*, 659. See Peter D. Olch, "William S. Halsted and Local Anesthesia: Contributions and Complications," *Anesthesiology*, 1975, *42*, 479–86; and Wilder Penfield, "Halsted of Johns Hopkins: The Man and His Problems as Described in the Secret Records of William Osler," *JAMA*, 1969, *210*, 2214–18.

15. John Parascandola, *The Development of American Pharmacology: John J. Abel*

and the Shaping of a Discipline (Baltimore: Johns Hopkins University Press, 1992), p. 59.

16. Ann Oakley, *The Captured Womb: A History of the Medical Care of Pregnant Women* (Oxford: Basil Blackwell, 1984), pp. 98–105.

17. Maynard Ladd, "Gastric Motility in Infants as Shown by the Roentgen Ray," *Am. J. Dis. Child.*, 1913, *5*, 345–58; Godfrey R. Pisek and Leon Theodore LeWald, "The Further Study of the Anatomy and Physiology of the Infant Stomach Based on Serial Roentgenograms," ibid., 1913, *6*, 232–44; Alfred Hess, "Use of Bismuth Pills in Fluoroscopic Examination of the Infant's Stomach," ibid., 1915, *9*, 461–77; Charles Hendee Smith and Leon Theodore LeWald, "Influence of Posture on Digestion in Infancy," ibid., 1915, *9*, 261–82.

18. Charles E. Rosenberg, *The Care of Strangers: The Rise of America's Hospital System* (New York: Basic Books, 1987), p. 5.

19. Michael Foster, "Scientific Use of Hospitals," *Nineteenth Century*, 1901, *49*, 57–63.

20. A. McGehee Harvey, *Science at the Bedside: Clinical Research in American Medicine, 1905–1945* (Baltimore: Johns Hopkins University Press, 1981), pp. 78–85.

21. Herbert O. Collins, "The Relation of the Hospital Superintendent to Research Work," *Trans. Am. Hosp. Assoc.*, 1917, *19*, 233.

22. Quoted in Warner, *Therapeutic Perspective*, p. 191.

23. Thomas N. Bonner, *American Doctors and German Universities* (Lincoln: University of Nebraska Press, 1963), pp. 104–5. Alexander M. Kidd, "Limits of the Rights of a Person to Consent to Experimentation on Himself," *Science*, 1953, *117*, 211–12.

24. J. M. T. Finney, *A Surgeon's Life* (New York: G. P. Putnam's Sons, 1940), p. 127. For the defense of a European physician accused of mistreating a hospital patient, see "An Alleged Hospital Scandal," *Phila. Med. J.*, 1900, *6*, 236.

25. Gladys-Marie Fry, *Night Riders in Black Folk History* (Knoxville: University of Tennessee Press, 1975), p. 172.

26. "Hospital Experiments," *Outlook*, 1900, *65*, 889–90.

27. For the report, see Roberts Bartholow, "Experimental Investigations into the Functions of the Human Brain," *Am. J. Med. Sci.*, 1874, *67*, 305–13. Quote is from pages 310–11.

28. David Ferrier, "Bartholow's Experiments on the Human Brain," *London Med. Rec.*, 1874, *2*, 285–86.

29. "Human Vivisection," *Cincinnati Med. News*, 1874, *3*, 385. For a discussion of Bartholow's experiments in the context of nineteenth-century cerebral localization studies, see James P. Morgan, "The First Electrical Stimulation of the Human Brain," *J. Hist. Med.*, 1982, *37*, 51–64.

30. Roberts Bartholow, "Experiments on the Functions of the Human Brain," *Br. Med. J.*, 1874, *1*, 727.

31. "Letter from a Hospital Patient Not of the Good Samaritan Hospital," *Cincinnati Med. News*, 1874, *3*, 234–35.

32. "Dr. Bartholow's Experiments," *Br. Med. J.*, 1874, *1*, 723.

33. Charles Francis Withington, *The Relation of Hospitals to Medical Education*

(Boston: Cupples, Upham, 1886), p. 16. For biographical information, see Walter P. Bowers, "Obituary: Charles Francis Withington," *Boston Med. Surg. J.*, 1917, *176*, 793–95.

34. Withington, *Relation of Hospitals to Medical Education*, p. 18.

35. This incident is discussed in Richard D. French, *Antivivisection and Medical Science in Victorian Society* (Princeton: Princeton University Press, 1975), pp. 320–22. For criticism, see Arthur Westcott, "The Danger to Hospital Patients in the Practice of Vivisection," *J. Zoophily*, 1896, *5*, 135–37; "Human Vivisection," *Our Fellow Creatures*, 1899, *7*, 132.

36. Withington, *Relation of Hospitals to Medical Education*, p. 17.

37. "The Trials of the Experimental Therapeutist," *Therapeutic Gazette*, 1884, *8*, 30–32.

38. John V. Shoemaker, "Address on Practical Medicine," *JAMA*, 1883, *2*, 518–19.

39. Victor Cornil, "Sur les greffes et inoculations de cancer," *Bulletin de l'Académie de Médecine*, 1891, *25*, 906–9.

40. Susan E. Lederer, "The Cancer-Grafting Scandal: Etiology and Ethics in the Late Nineteenth Century," unpublished manuscript.

41. "Grafting Cancer in the Human Subject," *JAMA*, 1891, *17*, 233–34. See also "Human Vivisection," *Med. News*, 1891, *59*, 137; "Cancer-grafting," *Med. Rec.*, 1891, *40*, 338; and "The Cancer-grafting Scandal," *Br. Med. J.*, 1891, *2*, 495.

42. Nicholas Senn, "A Plea for the International Study of Carcinoma," *JAMA*, 1906, *46*, 1255.

43. See "Experiments on Dying Patients," *New York Times*, 8 July 1891, p. 3; and "Cancer-grafting Operations," ibid., 21 July 1891, p. 5.

44. "Inoculation of Cancerous Matter," *Lancet*, 1891, *2*, 204.

45. Claude Bernard, *An Introduction to the Study of Experimental Medicine* (New York: Dover, 1957), p. 101.

46. Ibid., p. 102; and Jack Kevorkian, "A Brief History of Experimentation on Condemned and Executed Humans," *J. Nat. Med. Assoc.*, 1985, *77*, 215–26.

47. "Inoculation of Cancer," *Boston Med. Surg. J.*, 1891, *125*, 200–201.

48. Ibid.

49. William B. Coley, "The Treatment of Malignant Tumors by Repeated Inoculations of Erysipelas," *Am. J. Med. Sci.*, 1893, *105*, 492.

50. R. H. Chittenden and J. P. C. Foster, "Some Results of the Treatment of Tuberculosis with Koch's Lymph," *Am. J. Med. Sci.*, 1891, *102*, 1–18.

51. "Observations on Koch's Lymph," *JAMA*, 1891, *16*, 788–90.

52. "Official Regulations as to Tuberculin in Germany and Italy," *JAMA*, 1891, *16*, 492.

53. Withington, *Relation of Hospitals to Medical Education*, p. 17.

54. James W. Etheridge, "The Relative Indication for Cesarean Section," *Am. J. Obstet.*, 1888, *21*, 754.

55. Stanley Joel Reiser, "Words as Scalpels: Transmitting Evidence in the Clinical Dialogue," *Ann. Int. Med.*, 1980, *92*, 837.

56. Worthington Hooker quoted in Ruth Faden and Tom Beauchamp, *The History and Theory of Informed Consent* (Oxford: Oxford University Press, 1986), p. 71. See also Donald E. Konold, *A History of American Medical Ethics, 1847–1912* (Madison: Wisconsin State Historical Society, 1962), pp. 43–55.

57. Richard C. Cabot, "The Use of Truth and Falsehood in Medicine: An Experimental Study," *Am. Med.*, 1903, *5*, 344–49. See Chester Burns, "Richard Clarke Cabot (1868–1939) and the Reformation in American Medical Ethics," *Bull. Hist. Med.*, 1977, *51*, 353–68; and Paul D. White, "Richard Clarke Cabot," *N. Eng. J. Med.*, 1939, *220*, 1049–52.

58. Faden and Beauchamp, *History and Theory of Informed Consent*, p. 76. Also see Jay Katz, *The Silent World of Doctor and Patient* (New York: Free Press, 1984).

59. Thorne M. Carpenter and John R. Murlin, "The Energy Metabolism of Mother and Child Just Before and Just After Birth," *Arch. Int. Med.*, 1911, *7*, 184–222.

60. Albert Bernheim, "Movements of Intestines," *JAMA*, 1901, *36*, 429–31.

61. M. F. Engman, Rudolph Buhman, F. D. Gorham, and R. H. Davis, "A Study of the Spinal Fluid in One Hundred Cases of Syphilis," *JAMA*, 1913, *61*, 735–38.

62. Claude A. Smith, "Uncinariasis in the South, With Special Reference to Mode of Infection," *JAMA*, 1904, *43*, 592–97.

63. Francis Gano Benedict and Victor Carl Myers, "The Elimination of Creatine," *Am. J. Phys.*, 1907, *18*, 406–12.

64. Otto Folin and Philip A. Shaffer, "On Phosphate Metabolism," *Am. J. Phys.*, 1902, *7*, 135–51.

65. John Albert Marshall, "The Neutralizing Power of Saliva in Its Relation to Dental Caries," *Am. J. Phys.*, 1915, *36*, 260–79; and "The Salivary Factor and Its Relation to Dental Caries and Immunity in Dementia Praecox and Epilepsy," *Am. J. Phys.*, 1916, *40*, 2.

66. Wilder Tileston and C. W. Comfort, "The Total Nonprotein Nitrogen and the Urea of the Blood," *Am. J. Dis. Child.*, 1915, *10*, 278–79.

67. Susan E. Lederer, "Orphans As Guinea Pigs: American Children and Medical Experimenters, 1890–1930," in *In the Name of the Child: Health and Social Policy, 1870–1940*, ed. Roger Cooter (London: Routledge, 1992), pp. 96–123.

68. See, for example: T. J. Mahoney, "Suggestions on Rights and Liabilities of Surgeons," *JAMA*, 1900, *34*, 973–75; "The Consent of the Patients or Relatives to Operation," *Am. Med.*, 1903, *6*, 127; John Franklin Shields, "As to the Necessity of Consent to Render Surgical Operations Lawful," *Ann. Surg.*, 1905, *42*, 762–73; W. S. Wermuth, "Necessity of Consent to Operations," *JAMA*, 1913, *61*, 383–85; and Lorenzo D. Bulette, "Performing An Operation without Consent," *Int. Clin.*, 1914, *24*, 277–88.

69. John A. Hornsby and R. E. Schmidt, *The Modern Hospital* (Philadelphia: W. B. Saunders, 1913), p. 464.

70. Martin S. Pernick, *A Calculus of Suffering* (New York: Columbia University Press, 1985), pp. 208–16.

71. The *Schloendorf* decision is abstracted in Jay Katz, *Experimentation with Human Beings* (New York: Russell Sage Foundation, 1972), pp. 526–29.

72. Hornsby and Schmidt, *The Modern Hospital*, p. 507.

73. See "The Legal Aspect of Autopsies," *Boston Med. Surg. J.*, 1896, *134*, 272–73, for medical uncertainty over which next of kin should be consulted. See George H. Weinmann, "A Survey of the Law Concerning Dead Human Bodies," *Bulletin of the National Research Council*, 1929, *73*, 1–199.

74. Reports of suits for damages for human vivisection appeared in the Hearst press; see "Sues City for Lost Health," *New York Times*, 11 May 1913, p. 10. See George J. Annas, "The Nuremberg Code in U.S. Courts: Ethics versus Expediency," in *The Nazi Doctors and the Nuremberg Code: Human Rights in Human Experimentation* George J. Annas and Michael A. Grodin, eds. (New York: Oxford University Press, 1992), pp. 202–3. Also see Harry J. Keaton, "Torts: Physicians and Surgeons: Malpractice: Liability for Medical Experimentation," *Calif. Law Rev.*, 1952, *40*, 159–65.

75. "Koch's Method in Pulmonary Tuberculosis," *JAMA*, 1891, *16*, 105–8.

76. Faden and Beauchamp, *History and Theory of Informed Consent*, p. 100; Charles J. Weigel, "Medical Malpractice in America's Middle Years," *Texas Rep. Biol. Med.*, 1974, *32*, 191–205; and Katz, *Experimentation with Human Beings*, pp. 527–28.

77. T. M. Vogelsang, "A Serious Sentence Passed against the Discoverer of the Leprosy Bacillus (Gerhard Armauer Hansen) in 1880," *Med. Hist.*, 1963, *7*, 182–86; and Knut Blom, "Armauer Hansen and Human Leprosy Transmission," *Int. J. Lepr.*, 1973, *41*, 199–207.

78. See "Experiments on Human Beings," *JAMA*, 1900, *34*, 1358–59; and Barbara Elkeles, "Medizinische Menschenversuche gegen Ende des 19. Jahrhunderts und der Fall Neisser," *Medizin Historisches Journal*, 1985, *20*, 135–48.

79. "Damage Suit for Inoculation of Malaria," *JAMA*, 1903, *40*, 1290.

80. Isaac Abt, "Spontaneous Hemorrhages in Newborn Children," *JAMA*, 1903, *40*, 290.

81. See A. J. Rongy, "The Use of Fetal Serum to Cause the Onset of Labor," *Am. J. Obstet.*, 1912, *66*, 9–10.

82. Pernick, *A Calculus of Suffering*, p. 277.

83. Joseph William Stickler, "Some Achievements of Koch's 'Lymph,'" *NY Med. J.*, 1891, *53*, 99.

84. "Recent Experiments with the Pneumococcus of Pneumonia and Its Toxine and Antitoxine," *Boston Med. Surg. J.*, 1891, *125*, 530–31.

85. Francis G. Benedict, L. E. Emmes, and J. A. Riche, "The Influence of the Preceding Diet on the Respiratory Quotient after Active Digestion Has Ceased," *Am. J. Phys.*, 1911, *27*, p. 391.

86. Nancy Stepan, "The Interplay between Socio-Economic Factors and Medical Science: Yellow Fever Research, Cuba and the United States," *Soc. Stud. Sci.*, 1978, *8*, 397–423.

87. James Carroll to Surgeon General Sternberg, 29 Aug. 1906, Hench Collection, UVA, box 28, f. 40.

88. See Altman's discussion of the "myth of Walter Reed" in *Who Goes First?*, pp. 128–58.

89. Walter Reed to Jefferson R. Kean, 25 Sept. 1900, Hench Collection, UVA, box 21, f. 25.

90. Quoted in William B. Bean, "Walter Reed and the Ordeal of Human Experimentation," *Bull. Hist. Med.*, 1977, *51*, 87.

91. Informed Consent Agreement between Antonio Benigno and Walter Reed, 26 Nov. 1900, Hench Collection, UVA, box 70, f. 4.

92. Martha L. Sternberg, *George Miller Sternberg: A Biography* (Chicago: American Medical Association, 1920); and Edgar Erskine Hume, "Sternberg's Centenary, 1838–1938," *The Military Surgeon*, 1939, *84*, 420–28.

93. G. M. Sternberg to Agramonte, 14 May 1900, Hench Collection, UVA, box 20, f. 15.

94. George M. Sternberg, "Further Experiments with the Micrococcus of Gonorroeal Pus—'Gonococcus' of Neisser," *Med. News*, 1884, *45*, 426–29.

95. Ibid., p. 428.

96. Margaret H. Warner, "Hunting the Yellow Fever Germ: The Principle and Practice of Etiological Proof in Late Nineteenth Century America," *Bull. Hist. Med.*, 1985, *59*, 361–82. Warner minimizes the impact of Sanarelli's human experiments.

97. George M. Sternberg, "The Bacillus Icteroides (Sanarelli) and Bacillus X (Sternberg), *Trans. Assoc. Am. Physicians*, 1898, *13*, 70–71. See also discussion by William Osler and V. C. Vaughan on "The Bacillus Icteroides (Sanarelli) and Bacillus X (Sternberg)," *Trans. Assoc. Am. Physicians*, 1898, *13*, 61–72.

98. "Pan-American Medical Conference," *JAMA*, 1901, *36*, 461–62, included Louis Perna's criticism of the human experiments in yellow fever transmission. For an editorial defending the use of human volunteers, see "The Etiology of Yellow Fever," ibid., 446–47.

99. Quoted in Bean, "Walter Reed," p. 86.

100. George M. Sternberg, "Yellow Fever and Mosquitoes," *Popular Science Monthly*, 1901, *59*, 233.

101. "Horrendo . . . si es Cierto," *La discusión*, 21 Nov. 1900, Hench Collection, UVA, box 22, f. 12. See also William B. Bean, *Walter Reed: A Biography* (Charlottesville: University Press of Virginia, 1982), p. 147.

102. See "Yellow Fever Experiments in Cuba," *Br. Med. J.*, 1901, *2*, 638–39; "The Yellow Fever Experiments in Cuba," *JAMA*, 1901, *37*, 839–40; and "Second Victim of a Mosquito," *New York Times*, 20 Aug. 1901. See Harry F. Dowling, "Human Experimentation in Infectious Disease," *JAMA*, 1966, *198*, 997–99.

103. W. Reed and J. Carroll, "The Etiology of Yellow Fever," *Am. Med.*, 1902, *3*, 301.

104. See "Credit Due American Investigators," *JAMA*, 1904, *42*, 39; and for Reed as model, Walter D. Macaw, "Walter Reed," *Popular Science Monthly*, 1904, *65*, 262–68.

105. Gerald L. Geison, "Pasteur's Work on Rabies: Reexamining the Ethical Issues," *Hastings Cent. Rep.*, 1978, *8*, 26–33.

106. "Garnault Here," *JAMA*, 1903, *40*, 1151. Fortunately, Garnault's "robust

health" saved him from disease. See Barbara G. Rosenkrantz, "The Trouble with Bovine Tuberculosis," *Bull. Hist. Med.*, 1985, *59*, 155–75.

107. See "Dr. Barney May Be Prosecuted," *New York World*, 11 Nov. 1901; "No Peril Feared in Tuberculosis Test," and "Unwarrantable Human Experimentation," *New York Herald*, 12 Nov. 1901; "Health Board Won't Meddle," *New York Sun*, 12 Nov. 1901; "Dr. Barney Won't Be Arrested Yet," *New York World*, 12 Nov. 1901.

108. The *New York Herald* reported King's suicide by poisoning in July 1902; the *New York Journal* reported that Barney was sued for libel by the *Brooklyn Eagle* and incarcerated due to lack of bail money; see "A Celebrated Case," *Animals' Defender*, 1902, *7*, 12–13.

109. "A Questionable Editorial," *New York World*, 12 Nov. 1901, p. 8.

110. "Human and Bovine Tuberculosis," *JAMA*, 1902, *38*, 39; and for Dr. Barney's reply, see "Correspondence: Human and Bovine Tuberculosis," *JAMA*, 1902, *38*, 187–88.

111. "The Question of Voluntary Human Vivisection," *Am. Med.*, 1902, *3*, 253.

112. For newspaper accounts, see "Wants to be Vivisected," *New York Tribune*, 7 Feb. 1902; "Fantastic at Best," ibid., 8 Feb. 1902; and "Accept Russell's Offer," ibid., 8 Feb. 1902.

113. D. W. Cathell and William T. Cathell, *Book on the Physician Himself* (Philadelphia: F. A. Davis Co., 1906), p. 199.

114. Edward Hornibrook, "The Art of Medicine," *JAMA*, 1906, *47*, 817–19.

115. Grover Cleveland, "The Plea of the Patient," *Albany Medical Annals*, 1906, *27*, 156.

116. "Mrs. Phelps Ward on Vivisection," in *Vivisection* (Bristol: British Union for the Abolition of Vivisection, 1901), p. 2.

Chapter Two

1. Albert T. Leffingwell, "Scientific Assassination," *Twenty-first Annual Report of the American Humane Association*, 1897, pp. 38–39.

2. Ibid., p. 40.

3. James Turner's history of Anglo-American animal protection and antivivisection does not discuss human vivisection; see his *Reckoning with the Beast* (Baltimore: Johns Hopkins University Press, 1980). For discussion of antivivisection in the history of human experimentation, see Gert H. Brieger, "Human Experimentation: History," in *Encyclopedia of Bioethics*, ed. Warren T. Reich (New York: Free Press, 1978), pp. 684–92.

4. W. Bruce Fye, *The Development of American Physiology: Scientific Medicine in the Nineteenth Century* (Baltimore: Johns Hopkins University Press, 1987), pp. 33–34.

5. Zulma Steele, *Angel in Top Hat* (New York: Harper & Brothers, 1942), pp. 36–42.

6. Roswell C. McCrea, *The Humane Movement: A Descriptive Survey* (New York: Columbia University Press, 1910), pp. 147–56.

7. Lela B. Costin, "Unraveling the Mary Ellen Legend: Origins of the 'Cruelty' Movement," *Social Service Review*, 1991, *65*, 203–23.

8. Mary Ellen's story ended happily; see Stephen Lazoritz, "Whatever Happened to Mary Ellen?" *Child Abuse Negl.*, 1990, *14*, 143–49.

9. For the history of the influential Massachusetts society, see Linda Gordon, *Heroes of Their Own Lives: The Politics and History of Family Violence, Boston 1880–1960* (New York: Viking, 1988), esp. pp. 34–35, for links to the SPCA.

10. McCrea, *The Humane Movement*, p. 137.

11. Ibid., pp. 14–15.

12. Turner, *Reckoning with the Beast*, p. 37.

13. Ibid., pp. 37–38.

14. "Biography of Henry Bergh," app. 1 in McCrea, *The Humane Movement*, p. 151.

15. See "Notes and News," *Science*, 1886, *8*, 99.

16. Fye, *Development of American Physiology*, pp. 33–34.

17. For early experiments, see Edward C. Atwater, " 'Squeezing Mother Nature': Experimental Physiology in the United States before 1870," *Bull. Hist. Med.*, 1978, *52*, 313–35.

18. Address at Clinton Hall, 8 Feb. 1866, Edward P. Buffet Summary, vol. 4, ASPCA.

19. Frederick L. Holmes, "John Call Dalton," *Dictionary of Scientific Biography* (New York: Charles Scribner's Sons, 1978), vol. 15, suppl. 1, pp. 107–10; and John Harley Warner, "Physiology," in *The Education of American Physicians: Historical Essays*, ed. Ronald L. Numbers (Berkeley: University of California Press, 1980), p. 58.

20. Student to Henry Bergh, 17 Oct. 1867, Buffet Summary, ASPCA.

21. See Bergh to Flint, 19 Oct. 1867; Flint to Bergh, 25 Oct. 1867; and ASPCA annual report for year ending 30 Apr. 1868 in Edward P. Buffet Summary, vol. 4, ASPCA.

22. John C. Dalton, "Vivisection, What It Is and What It Has Accomplished," *Bull. NY Acad. Med.*, 1866–69, *3*, 159–98.

23. John C. Dalton, *Experimentation on Animals, as a Means of Knowledge in Physiology, Pathology, and Practical Medicine* (New York: F. W. Christern, 1875), pp. 29–41.

24. "Mr. Bergh and the Doctors," *NY Med. J.*, 1867, *5*, 71–80. See also G. Hamilton, "Thoughts upon Vivisection, with Reference to its Restriction by Legislative Action," *Trans. Coll. Phys. Phila.*, 1881, *3*, 103–19; and J. M. Beck, "The Legal Aspects of Vivisection," *Med. News*, 1890, *56*, 280–82.

25. *Sixteenth Annual Report of the American Humane Association* (Philadelphia, 1892), pp. 29–36.

26. Caroline Earle White, "The History of the Anti-Vivisection Movement," in *Proceedings of the International Anti-Vivisection and Animal Protection Congress* (New York: Tudor Press, [1914?]), pp. 25–35. For biographical material on White, see Sydney H. Coleman, *Humane Society Leaders in America* (Albany: American Humane Association, 1924), pp. 178–86; and McCrea, *The Humane Movement*, pp. 221–22.

27. White, "History of the Anti-Vivisection Movement," p. 31.

28. William J. Shultz, *The Humane Movement in the United States, 1910–1922* (1924; New York: AMS Press, 1968), pp. 141–61.

29. Coleman, *Humane Society Leaders*, p. 181.

30. "Kindness to Animals," *J. Zoophily*, 1899, *8*, 27.

31. "Mrs. C. E. White, Humanitarian, Dies," *Philadelphia Inquirer*, 7 Sept. 1916.

32. "The South Omaha Bull Fights," *J. Zoophily*, 1901, *10*, 90.

33. F. Morse Hubbard, "Prevention of Cruelty to Animals in the States of Illinois, Colorado, and California," *Proc. Acad. Pol. Sci.*, 1916, *6*, 80; and "Water for Horses at Police Stations," *J. Zoophily*, 1914, *23*, 120.

34. "Extracts from the Ninth Annual Report of the Department of Mercy of the National Woman's Christian Temperance Union," *J. Zoophily*, 1899, *8*, 136. See Robin W. Doughty, *Feather Fashions and Bird Preservation* (Berkeley: University of California Press, 1975), pp. 188–89.

35. Archie Binns, *Mrs. Fiske and the American Theatre* (New York: Crown, 1955), p. 271.

36. C. E. White, "Notes," *J. Zoophily*, 1913, *22*, 53.

37. Binns, *Mrs. Fiske*, p. 345. For humanifur, see "Mrs. Robert P. Logan," *The Starry Cross*, 1929, *37*, 37; and "Humanifur Exhibit," ibid., p. 134.

38. *Report of the American Humane Association on Vivisection in America* (Cambridge, Mass.: University Press, 1895), p. 8. See Susan E. Lederer, "The Controversy over Animal Experimentation in America, 1880–1914," in *Vivisection in Historical Perspective*, ed. Nicolaas Rupke, (London: Croom Helm, 1987), pp. 236–58.

39. *Vivisection in America*, p. 25.

40. Some recent writers have followed this example; see Thomas A. Woolsey and Robert E. Burke, with Susan Sauer, "The Playwright, the Practitioner, the Politician, the President, and the Pathologist: A Guide to the 1900 Senate Document Titled *Vivisection*," *Perspect. Biol. Med.*, 1987, *30*, 235–58.

41. "Anti-Vivisection Extremism," *Med. Rec.*, 1896, *50*, 54. See also "The New York Quakers on Vivisection," *NY Med. J.*, 1899, *69*, 786.

42. McCrea, *The Humane Movement*, p. 123.

43. That few records exist is not surprising; lacking large endowments, these societies moved a great deal. See Richard D. French, *Antivivisection and Medical Science in Victorian Society* (Princeton: Princeton University Press, 1975), pp. 221–22, 239–46, for problems assessing membership in British antivivisection societies.

44. See *Annual Report*, 1935–36, New England Anti-Vivisection Society.

45. The eminent English historian Edward Lecky, quoted in "Mr. Lecky on Women as Antivivisectionists," *Boston Med. Surg. J.*, 1896, *135*, 150–51.

46. Stanton, quoted in the *Rochester World*; see "Passing Down the Vale under a Cloud," *Anti-Vivisection*, 1896–97, *4*, 19.

47. Charles Dana, "The Zoophil-Psychosis," *Med. Rec.*, 1909, *75*, 381–83.

48. James P. Warbasse, *The Conquest of Disease Through Animal Experimentation* (New York: D. Appleton, 1910), p. 159.

49. Amanda M. Hale, "The Correlated Duties of the Medical Profession and the Humane Public as Regards Vivisection," *J. Zoophily*, 1898, *7*, 22.

50. Regina Markell Morantz-Sanchez, *Sympathy and Science* (New York: Oxford University Press, 1985), p. 191.

51. Elizabeth Blackwell, "Erroneous Method in Medical Education," *Essays in Medical Sociology*, 2 vols., (New York: Arno, 1972), vol. 2, p. 43.

52. Morantz-Sanchez, *Sympathy and Science*, p. 191.

53. Coral Lansbury, "Gynaecology, Pornography, and the Antivivisection Movement," *Victorian Studies*, 1985, *28*, 413–37; and Lansbury, *The Old Brown Dog: Women, Workers, and Vivisection in Edwardian England* (Madison: University of Wisconsin Press, 1985), p. x.

54. Mary Ann Elston, "Women and Anti-Vivisection in Victorian England, 1870–1900," in Rupke, *Vivisection in Historical Perspective*, pp. 259–94.

55. Carol F. Kessler, *Elizabeth Stuart Phelps* (Boston: Twayne, 1982), p. 111.

56. John R. Murlin to the Hon. Daniel O'Mara, 14 Aug. 1934, George Hoyt Whipple Papers, UR, box 2, f. 12.

57. See Coleman, *Humane Society Leaders*, pp. 182–83.

58. Thomas Timmins, *The History of the Founding, Aims, and Growth of the American Bands of Mercy* (Boston: Massachusetts Society for the Prevention of Cruelty to Animals, n.d.).

59. "Mercy," *Union Signal*, 29 Nov. 1906, p. 14.

60. See Ruth Bordin, *Woman and Temperance: The Quest for Power and Liberty, 1873–1900* (Philadelphia: Temple University Press, 1981), pp. 98, 109.

61. For Mary Hanchett Hunt, see Philip J. Pauly, "The Struggle for Ignorance about Alcohol: American Physiologists, Wilbur Olin Atwater, and the Woman's Christian Temperance Union," *Bull. Hist. Med.*, 1990, *64*, 366–92.

62. Mary F. Lovell, "Humane Education," *Union Signal*, 13 Aug. 1899, p. 5. For 1923, see Shultz, *Humane Movement in the U.S.*, p. 130.

63. See David I. Macleod, *Building Character in the American Boy: The Boy Scouts, the YMCA, and Their Forerunners, 1870–1920* (Madison: University of Wisconsin Press, 1983).

64. Shultz, *Humane Movement in the U.S.*, p. 132.

65. Virginia Fairchild-Allen, "Don't Allow Boys to Destroy Life," *Anti-Vivisection*, 1897, *4*, 153.

66. "The Little Boy Who Never Grew Up," *Life*, 1911, *57*, 534.

67. Mary F. Lovell, "The World's Great Object Lesson," *Union Signal*, 30 June 1898, p. 4.

68. See Lederer, "The Controversy over Animal Experimentation in America, 1800–1914," pp. 241–44.

69. See Lloyd G. Stevenson, "Science down the Drain," *Bull. Hist. Med.*, 1955, *29*, 1–26.

70. Amanda M. Hale, "Is Tuberculosis Contagious?" *J. Zoophily*, 1899, *8*, 113–14.

71. See Albert Leffingwell, *The Vivisection Question*, 2nd ed. (Chicago: Vivisection Reform Society, 1907), pp. 176–80.

72. See testimony of Matthew Woods, M.D., in *Vivisection: Hearing before the Senate Committee on the District of Columbia, February 21, 1900, on the Bill (S. 34) For the*

Further Prevention of Cruelty to Animals in the District of Columbia (Washington, D.C.: Government Printing Office, 1900), p. 16.

73. The source of this quotation is J. Bentham, *An Introduction to the Principles of Morals and Legislation* (Oxford: Clarendon, 1907), p. 311. See also Nicolaas Rupke, "Pro-Vivisection in England in the Early 1880s: Arguments and Motives," in Rupke, *Vivisection in Historical Perspective*, pp. 188–213.

74. Statement by David H. Cochran in *Vivisection: Hearing before the Senate Committee, 1900*, p. 17. Leffingwell credited Cochran with changing his mind about the limited utility of vivisection.

75. "President Eliot of Harvard and Anti-Vivisection," *Med. News*, 1900, *76*, 832–33; "Legislation Against Medical Discovery," *Popular Science Monthly*, 1900, *57*, 436.

76. See "The Screamer," *Our Fellow Creatures*, 1900, *8*, 398.

77. See *Catalogue of the Exhibit American Anti-Vivisection Society* (Philadelphia), pamphlet in Frederic S. Lee Papers, Columbia University.

78. See Frank Luther Mott, *A History of American Magazines: 1885–1905* (Cambridge: Harvard University Press, 1957), pp. 556–68.

79. See Harvey W. Wiley, letter to the editor, *JAMA*, 1918, *71*, 1510–11. For cartoons, see *Life*, 1901, *54*, 52; 1910, *55*, 966–67; and 1914, *63*, 264. Catcarver Jones appeared in *Life*, 1913, *61*, 274.

80. Turner develops Victorian attitudes toward pain in *Reckoning with the Beast*, pp. 79–84; see also T. J. Jackson Lears, *No Place of Grace: Antimodernism and the Transformation of American Culture 1880–1920* (New York: Pantheon, 1981), pp. 45–46.

81. William James, *The Varieties of Religious Experience* (New York: Collier Books, 1961), p. 239.

82. Harold Lief and Renée Fox, "Training for 'Detached Concern' in Medical Students," in *The Psychological Basis of Medical Practice*, ed. Harold Lief, Victor Lief, and Nina Lief (New York: Harper & Row, 1963), pp. 21–22. See also Lansbury, *Old Brown Dog*, p. 178.

83. See "Vivisection Legislation," *New York Herald*, 18 Apr. 1908 (in Newspaper Clipping Book, 600–1, RUA). On the behavior of University of Michigan medical students and "hideous performances" with cadavers, see "Where Shall Our Boys Be Educated?" *Anti-Vivisection*, 1897, *4*, 30–31; "Ball-Playing with Corpses," ibid., 1895–96, *3*, 10.

84. Cleland K. Nelson, *Anti-Vivisection*, 1897, *4*, 58–59.

85. Keith Thomas, *Man and the Natural World: A History of the Modern Sensibility* (New York: Pantheon, 1983), pp. 294–95.

86. Turner, *Reckoning with the Beast*, p. 134.

87. This issue also arose at Britain's parliamentary hearings on vivisection; see Lloyd G. Stevenson, "On the Supposed Exclusion of Butchers and Surgeons from Jury Duty," *J. Hist. Med.*, 1954, *8*, 235–38.

88. "Mrs. Phelps Ward on Vivisection," in *Vivisection* (Bristol: British Union for the Abolition of Vivisection, 1901), p. 4. The line comes from the poem, "In the

Children's Hospital," in *The Poems of Alfred Lord Tennyson* (New York: Thomas Y. Crowell Co., 1897), pp. 569–72.

89. Murders by a Dr. Graves in Providence, a Dr. Buchanan in New York, a Dr. Cream in Canada, and by medical students in New York and California were reported in *Anti-Vivisection*, 1897, *4*, 45.

90. D. W. Cathell and William T. Cathell, *Book on the Physician Himself*, rev. ed. (Philadelphia: F. A. Davis Co., 1906), p. 142.

91. Richard H. Shryock, "Freedom and Interference in Medicine," *Ann. Am. Acad. Pol. Soc. Sci.*, 1938, *200*, 32–59. Bernhard J. Stern, *Social Factors in Medical Progress* (New York: Columbia University Press, 1927), pp. 34–43.

92. George B. Jenkins, "The Legal Status of Dissecting," *Anat. Rec.*, 1913, *7*, 387–99. David C. Humphrey, "Dissection and Discrimination: The Social Origins of Cadavers in America, 1760–1915," *Bull. NY Acad. Med.*, 1973, *49*, 819–27.

93. J. M. Emmert, "State Medicine, Past Present Future," *JAMA*, 1902, *36*, 1573.

94. Martin S. Pernick, "Back from the Grave: Recurring Controversies over Defining and Diagnosing Death in History," in *Death: Beyond Whole-Brain Criteria*, ed. Richard M. Zaner (Dordrecht, Netherlands: Kluwer Academic, 1988), pp. 17–74, esp. p. 47. Also see Marc Alexander, " 'The Rigid Embrace of the Narrow House': Premature Burial and the Signs of Death," *Hastings Cent. Rep.*, 1980, *10*, 25–31.

95. George T. Angell, "Burial of the Supposed Dead," *Our Dumb Animals*, 1896, *28*, 92. Also see H. Gerald Chapin, "The Proposed Law to Prevent Premature Burial," *Medico-Legal Journal*, 1898–99, *16*, 1–9.

96. "The Growing Practice of Premature Burial," *Current Literature*, 1907, *43*, 680–82; for physicians' responses, see "Premature Burial," *JAMA*, 1900, *34*, 115, and J. F. Baldwin, "Premature Burial," *Sci. Am.*, 1896, *75*, 315.

97. Beatrice Ethel Kidd and M. Edith Richards, *Hadwen of Gloucester: Man, Medico, Martyr* (London: John Murray, 1933), pp. 146–47.

98. E. E. Slosson, "The Relative Value of Life and Learning," *Independent* (New York), 12 Dec. 1895, p. 7; see Mary F. Lovell's correspondence with the *Independent*, which declined to publish her letter, in *J. Zoophily*, 1896, *5*, 15.

99. John S. Pyle, "A Plea for the Appropriation of Criminals, Condemned to Capital Punishment, to the Experimental Physiologist," *Tri-State Med. J.*, 1893–94, *1*, 5–11. See also Pyle, "Pneumonectomy, the Future Treatment of Incipient Pulmonary Tuberculosis," *NY Med. J.*, 1899, *69*, 817–19.

100. Pyle, "A Plea," p. 7; Pyle's article was apparently reprinted in both the *Peoria Med. Rec.* and the *American Journal of Politics*.

101. See also Jack Kevorkian, "A Brief History of Experimentation on Condemned and Executed Humans," *J. Nat. Med. Assoc.*, 1985, *77*, 215–26.

102. Rowlen corresponded with Mary Frances Lovell on the bill, see "Society News," *J. Zoophily*, 1894, *3*, 51. See "Vivisection of Criminals," *Our Fellow Creatures*, 1900, *8*, 83–84.

103. "Vivisection for Men Condemned to Death," *J. Zoophily*, 1903, *12*, 40–41; M. F. L. [Mary Frances Lovell], "What Are They?" *J. Zoophily*, 1902, *11*, 20–21; "The Vivisection of Criminals," *J. Zoophily*, 1903, *12*, 72–73.

104. See *J. Zoophily*, 1893, *2*, p. 34 for the *New York Recorder*'s advertisement for willing consumptives; *J. Zoophily*, 1894, *3*, 114 for an offer of $5,000 for an experimental operation. For report of a Cook County hospital that allegedly sold patients for experimentation before death, see "Threatened Fate of Hospital Patients," *Our Fellow Creatures*, 1898, *6*, 102.

105. Todd L. Savitt, "The Use of Blacks for Medical Experimentation and Demonstration in the Old South," *J. South. Hist.*, 1982, *48*, 331–48.

106. "The Fulfillment of Prophecy," *J. Zoophily*, 1894, *3*, 57; Mary F. Lovell, "The Bills in the Ohio Legislature for the Vivisection of Criminals," *Union Signal*, 29 Mar. 1894, p. 5.

107. William Williams Keen, "Our Recent Debts to Vivisection," *Popular Science Monthly*, 1885, *27*, 3.

108. Statement of Dr. Howard A. Kelly, *Vivisection: Hearing before the Senate Committee, 1900*, p. 64.

109. See "Albert Tracy Leffingwell," in *Physicians and Surgeons of the United States*, ed. Irving A. Watson (Concord, N.H.: Republican Press, 1896), pp. 56–57; obituary notice in *New York Times*, 2 Sept. 1916.

110. The Dansville Water Cure is discussed in Susan E. Cayleff, *Wash and Be Healed: The Water Cure Movement and Women's Health* (Philadelphia: Temple University Press, 1987), pp. 94–95. Elizabeth Fear married Albert Tracy Leffingwell (not Albert J.) in 1892. See Watson, *Physicians and Surgeons*, p. 57.

111. Dr. Hersey Locke to Frederic S. Lee, 24 Apr. 1908, Frederic S. Lee Papers, Columbia University.

112. Albert Leffingwell, *Illegitimacy and the Influence of Seasons upon Conduct* (London, 1891); Albert Tracy [pseudo.], *Rambles through Japan without a Guide* (London, 1892); Albert Leffingwell, *American Meat* (New York: Theo. E. Schulte, 1910).

113. See "Correspondence: The Vivisection Controversy," *Med. News*, 1895, *67*, 663–64.

114. See letters to the editor, Boston *Transcript*, 16 Oct. 1897 and 3 Nov. 1897; also reprinted in Leffingwell, *The Vivisection Question*, pp. 248–51.

115. For biographical material, see Pietro Ambrosioni, "Giuseppe Sanarelli," *Dictionary of Scientific Biography*, vol. 12 (New York: Charles Scribner's Sons, 1975), pp. 96–97.

116. G. Sanarelli, "A Lecture on Yellow Fever, with a Description of the Bacillus Icteroides," *Br. Med. J.*, 1897, *2*, 9. In antivivisectionist publications, the translation is always given as "the final collapse."

117. Quoted in Margaret Warner, "Hunting the Yellow Fever Germ: The Principle and Practice of Etiological Proof in Late Nineteenth-Century America," *Bull. Hist. Med.*, 1985, *59*, 373.

118. Leffingwell, "Scientific Assassination," p. 39.

Chapter Three

1. *Human Vivisection: Foundlings Cheaper than Animals* (Washington, D.C.: Humane Society, 1901).

2. See "Vivisection and Antivivisection," *Phila. Med. J.*, 1901, *7*, 370–74, esp. p. 370; the humane society used Jansen rather than Janson. For the original, see C. Janson, "Versuche zur Erlangung künstlicher Immunität bei Variola vaccina," *Centralbl. f. Bakteriol. u. Parasitenk.*, 1891, *10*, 40–45.

3. *Human Vivisection: Foundlings Cheaper than Animals.*

4. Paul Starr, *The Social Transformation of American Medicine* (New York: Basic, 1982).

5. See Patricia P. Gossel, "William Henry Welch and the Antivivisection Legislation in the District of Columbia, 1896–1900," *J. Hist. Med.*, 1985, *40*, 397–419; and Thomas A. Woolsey and Robert E. Burke, with Susan Sauer, "The Playwright, the Practitioner, the Politician, the President, and the Pathologist: A Guide to the 1900 Senate Document Titled *Vivisection*," *Perspect. Biol. Med.*, 1987, *30*, 235–58.

6. For the British act, see Richard D. French's indispensable *Antivivisection and Medical Science in Victorian Society* (Princeton: Princeton University Press, 1975).

7. See "Jacob H. Gallinger," in *Dictionary of American Temperance Biography*, ed. Mark E. Lender (Westport, Conn.: Greenwood, 1984), pp. 184–86; and "Jacob H. Gallinger," *Dictionary of American Biography*, vol. 7 (New York: Charles Scribner's Sons, 1931), pp. 112–13.

8. For criticism of Gallinger's medical qualifications, see "Old Doc Gallinger," *JAMA*, 1914, *62*, 1354–55.

9. William H. Welch, "Objections to the Antivivisection Bill Now Before the Senate of the United States," *JAMA*, 1898, *30*, 285.

10. See *Report and Hearing on S. 1552 For the Further Prevention of Cruelty to Animals in the District of Columbia*, Sen. Rep. 1049, 54th Cong., 1st sess., 26 May 1896.

11. Ibid.

12. The material conditions of research are astutely discussed in Adele Clarke, "Research Materials and Reproductive Science in the United States, 1910–1940," in *Physiology in the American Context, 1850–1940*, ed. Gerald L. Geison (Bethesda, Md.: American Physiological Society, 1987), pp. 323–50.

13. The extent to which the British act actually impeded physiologists has been disputed. Geison argues that the act was not a serious obstacle; see Gerald L. Geison, *Michael Foster and the Cambridge School of Physiology* (Princeton: Princeton University Press, 1978), p. 331. For a challenge to this interpretation, see Saul Benison, A. Clifford Barger, and Elin L. Wolfe, *Walter B. Cannon* (Cambridge: Harvard University Press, 1987), p. 445. I side with Geison, although it is clear that British investigators considered the act a serious obstacle to research.

14. Welch, "Objections to the Antivivisection Bill," p. 285.

15. See Kenneth M. Ludmerer, *Learning to Heal: The Development of American Medical Education* (New York: Basic Books, 1985); and Richard D. French, "Animal Experimentation: Historical Aspects," *Encyclopedia of Bioethics*, editor-in-chief, Warren T. Reich (New York: Free Press, 1978), vol. 1, pp. 75–79, esp. p. 77.

16. Ludmerer, *Learning to Heal*, pp. 47–53.

17. Bigelow was quoted in *Vivisection: Hearing before the Senate Committee on the District of Columbia, February 21, 1900, on the Bill (S. 34) For the Further Prevention of*

Cruelty to Animals in the District of Columbia (Washington, D.C.: Government Printing Office, 1900), p. 145.

18. Thomas S. Huddle, "Looking Backward: The 1871 Reforms at Harvard Medical School Reconsidered," *Bull. Hist. Med.*, 1991, *65*, 340–65.

19. Ludmerer, *Learning to Heal*, pp. 58–63; and *A Model of Its Kind*, vol. 1: *A Centennial History of Medicine at Johns Hopkins*, ed. A. McGehee Harvey, Gert H. Brieger, Susan L. Abrams, and Victor A. McKusick (Baltimore: Johns Hopkins University Press, 1989).

20. Abraham Flexner, *Medical Education in the United States and Canada* (Boston: Merrymount, 1910).

21. This is not to suggest that physiologists and bacteriologists used animal bodies in similar ways. Each of these disciplines, however, is constructed or inscribed in or on the bodies of animals; see Bruno Latour, *The Pasteurization of France* (Cambridge: Harvard University Press, 1988); and William Coleman, "The Cognitive Basis of the Discipline: Claude Bernard on Physiology," *Isis*, 1985, *76*, 49–70.

22. For American physicians and bacteriology, see William G. Rothstein, *American Physicians in the Nineteenth Century: From Sects to Science* (Baltimore: Johns Hopkins University Press, 1972), pp. 261–81.

23. John Harley Warner, *The Therapeutic Perspective: Medical Practice, Knowledge, and Identity in America, 1820–1885* (Cambridge: Harvard University Press, 1986), esp. pp. 272–73.

24. John Parascandola, *The Development of American Pharmacology: John J. Abel and the Shaping of a Discipline* (Baltimore: Johns Hopkins University Press, 1992), pp. 44–45, 50.

25. See "Experimental Medicine," *Med. Rec.*, 1883, *23*, 150.

26. Benison et al., *Walter B. Cannon*, pp. 172–75.

27. Welch served as a member of this committee; see Jonathan Dine Wirtschafter, "The Genesis and Impact of the Medical Lobby: 1898–1906," *J. Hist. Med.*, 1958, *13*, 15–49.

28. For heroic biography, see Simon Flexner and James Thomas Flexner, *William Henry Welch and the Heroic Age of American Medicine* (New York: Viking, 1941), pp. 254–62; and Donald Fleming, *William H. Welch and the Rise of Modern Medicine* (Boston: Little, Brown, 1954).

29. Welch began carrying manuscripts around in a trunk. This was one reason the journal was turned over to the Rockefeller Institute in 1905. See George W. Corner, *A History of the Rockefeller Institute* (New York: Rockefeller Institute Press, 1964), pp. 62–63.

30. See Flexner and Flexner, *William Henry Welch*, p. 257.

31. *Vivisection: Hearing before the Senate Committee, 1900*.

32. Keen published at least thirteen papers, two books, and eight letters to editors on animal experimentation; see Donald C. Geist, "The Writings of William W. Keen, M.D., Hon. F.R.C.S.: A Selected Annotated Bibliography," *Trans. Stud. Coll. Phys. Phila.*, 1976, *43*, 337–71.

33. William W. Keen, "Before and After Lister," in *Selected Papers and Addresses* (Philadelphia: George W. Jacobs, 1923), p. 173.

34. William Williams Keen, *Animal Experimentation and Medical Progress* (Boston: Houghton Mifflin, 1914), p. 287.

35. "Hampering Animal Experimentation," *JAMA*, 1912, *58*, 863; and Morris Joseph Clurman, "The Present Status of Vivisection in the Medical Profession," *NY Med. J.*, 1911, *94*, 865–73, esp. p. 868.

36. See W. H. Welch to Keen, 23 Jan. 1900, and 5 Feb. 1900, Keen Papers, CPP.

37. For a thorough analysis of the testimony at the 1900 hearing (although they misspell Henry Bergh's name), see Woolsey and Burke, "The Playwright, the Practitioner."

38. See Charles E. Rosenberg, *No Other Gods: On Science and American Social Thought* (Baltimore: Johns Hopkins University Press, 1976). On the popularization of science, see John C. Burnham, *How Superstition Won and Science Lost* (New Brunswick, N.J.: Rutgers University Press, 1987).

39. See G. Kendall, "Is the Cure of Disease the Highest Boon Modern Science Can Give Us?" *Our Fellow Creatures*, 1898, *6*, 162.

40. See David Rothman's perceptive discussion of the virtually indestructible optimism that imbued Progressive reformers, "The State as Parent: Social Policy in the Progressive Era," in *Doing Good: The Limits of Benevolence*, ed. Willard Gaylin et al. (New York: Pantheon, 1978), pp. 67–96.

41. For the "undue importance" accorded bacteriology, see Theophilus Parvin's 1891 presidential address to the American Academy of Medicine, *A Physician on Vivisection* (Cambridge, Mass.: J. Wilson & Son, 1895).

42. James Turner, *Reckoning with the Beast* (Baltimore: Johns Hopkins University Press, 1980), pp. 122–37.

43. Quoted in E. V. Wilcox, "The Anti-Vivisection Agitation," *J. Comp. Med. & Vet. Arch.*, 1898, *19*, 792.

44. Warner, *The Therapeutic Perspective*, p. 273.

45. "Practical Value of Bacteriological Examination of the Blood," *JAMA*, 1903, *41*, 500.

46. "The Etiology of Syphilis," *JAMA*, 1905, *45*, 108.

47. For the "disaster" of Koch's tuberculin, see John Madden, "The Limitations of Serum Therapy," *JAMA*, 1898, *30*, 1165. Tuberculin of course became an invaluable diagnostic tool; see Rothstein, *American Physicians*, pp. 269–70, and Edward Shapiro, "Robert Koch and His Tuberculin Fallacy," *Pharos*, 1983, *46*, 19–22.

48. See Woolsey and Burke, "The Playwright, the Practitioner," p. 252.

49. D. W. Cathell and William T. Cathell, *Book on the Physician Himself*, rev. ed. (Philadelphia: F. A. Davis Co., 1906), p. 144.

50. *Vivisection in the District of Columbia*, Sen. Doc. 78, 55th Cong., 3rd sess., 26 Jan. 1899, pp. 28–34.

51. George L. Fitch, "The Etiology of Leprosy," *Med. Rec.*, 1892, *42*, 293–303. Fitch's theory was not wholly eccentric; in 1886 the Royal College of Physicians

conducted a small survey about leprosy. Although twenty-one physicians believed there was no relation between syphilis and leprosy, twelve regarded the two diseases as intimately related. See "Notes and News," *Science*, 1886, *8*, 511.

52. Fitch was not the only physician to perform experiments with leprosy. See "Honolulu Letter," *Science*, 1886, *8*; 73–75; "The Inoculation of a Condemned Criminal," *Med. Rec.*, 1886, *29*, 449; and A. A. St. Maur Moritz, "Human Inoculation Experiments in Hawaii, including Notes on those of Arning and Fitch," *Int. J. Lepr.*, 1951, *19*, 203–15.

53. Henry J. Berkley, "Studies on the Lesions Induced by the Action of Certain Poisons on the Cortical Nerve Cell. Study VII: Poisoning with Preparations of the Thyroid Gland," *Bull. Johns Hopkins Hosp.*, 1897, *8*, 137–40.

54. Ibid., p. 138.

55. Hospitals had become increasingly concerned about legal requirements for consent to autopsy; see "The Legal Aspect of Autopsies," *Boston Med. Surg. J.*, 1896, *134*, 272–73.

56. Berkley, "Studies on Lesions," p. 139.

57. Arthur H. Wentworth, "Some Experimental Work on Lumbar Puncture of the Subarachnoid Space," *Boston Med. Surg. J.*, 1896, *135*, 132–36, 156–61.

58. Ibid., p. 133.

59. Ibid.

60. *Human Vivisection: A Statement and an Inquiry*, 3rd rev. ed. (American Humane Association, 1900).

61. George M. Searle, "Murder in the Name of Science," *Catholic World*, 1900, *70*, 493–504, and "Murder and Science," *JAMA*, 1900, *34*, 242; and *Human Vivisection: Foundlings Cheaper than Animals*.

62. *Vivisection: Hearing before the Senate Committee, 1900*, p. 32.

63. Osler's response seems disingenuous in light of Berkley's arrangement to teach Hopkins medical students at the Bay View asylum; see Alan M. Chesney, *The Johns Hopkins Hospital and the Johns Hopkins University School of Medicine: A Chronicle*, vol. 2, *1893–1905* (Baltimore: Johns Hopkins University Press, 1958), p. 84.

64. *Vivisection: Hearing before the Senate Committee, 1900*, pp. 64–65.

65. William Osler, *The Principles and Practice of Medicine*, 3rd ed., rev. (New York: Appleton, 1898), p. 183. Keen supplied Gallinger with this citation on 21 Mar. 1900, see Keen to Jacob H. Gallinger, Keen Papers, CPP.

66. "The Vivisection of Children," *The Animal's Defender*, 1903, *8*, 17–23.

67. The thirty-seven interruptions are by Woolsey and Burke's count (see "The Playwright, the Practitioner," p. 245); see also *Vivisection: Hearing before the Senate Committee, 1900*, p. 30.

68. See W. W. Keen, "Misstatements on Antivivisection," *JAMA*, 1901, *36*, 501–5. In response to Keen, the AHA published *The Reality of Human Vivisection: A Review* (Boston, 1901), and *Concerning Human Vivisection: A Controversy* (Washington, D.C.: American Humane Association, 1901); "Vivisection and Antivivisection," pp. 370–74.

69. See W. W. Keen, "Influence of Antivivisection on Character," *Boston Med. Surg. J.*, 1912, *166*, 651–58, 687–94, esp. p. 653.

70. Wilcox, "The Anti-Vivisection Agitation," p. 787.

71. Keen, "Misstatements on Antivivisection," p. 504.

72. *Human Vivisection: Foundlings Cheaper than Animals*, p. 1.

73. W. H. Welch to W. W. Keen, 13 Dec. 1900, William Henry Welch Papers, Johns Hopkins University.

74. Stuart explained that Leffingwell was one of his first acquaintances in Brooklyn. The two became very close, and in fact, Stuart served as the medical adviser for Leffingwell's wife during her confinement. For these reasons, Stuart asked Keen not to cite him as the source of information about Tracy, even though he shared Keen's opinion. See Francis H. Stuart to W. W. Keen, 4 Mar. 1901, 26 Apr. 1901, in Keen Papers, CPP.

75. *Dr. Keen and Human Vivisection* (pamphlet, n.d.).

76. W. W. Keen to W. H. Welch, 4 Mar. 1901, Keen Papers, CPP; for criticism of the anonymous review of Keen's letter, see George H. Simmons to James M. Brown, 13 May 1901, Keen Papers, CPP.

77. Welch shared this opinion. See W. H. Welch to W. W. Keen, 13 Dec. 1900, Keen Papers, CPP.

78. For the original paper, see Schreiber, "Ueber das Koch'sche Heilverfahren," *Dtsch. Med. Wochenschr.*, 1891, *17*, 306–9.

79. Keen, "Misstatements on Antivivisection," p. 504.

80. Wentworth, "Some Experimental Work," p. 136.

81. Keen, "Misstatements on Antivivisection," p. 503.

82. Ibid., p. 502.

83. "Vivisection and Antivivisection," p. 372, where Keen accuses the humane society of mutilating its own documents as well.

84. W. H. Welch to W. W. Keen, 21 Mar. 1900, Keen Papers, CPP.

85. Ibid.

86. William Mabon and Warren L. Babcock, "Thyroid Extract—A Review of the Results obtained in the Treatment of One Thousand Thirty-two Collected Cases of Insanity," *Am. J. Insanity*, 1899, *56*, 257–73.

87. W. H. Welch to W. W. Keen, 21 Mar. 1900.

88. Edward Berdoe, an English physician and antivivisectionist, criticized Berkley in the *Daily Chronicle* in September 1897. See "Experiments on Lunatics," *Br. Med. J.*, 1897, *2*, 728–29, and Berdoe's rejoinder, "Experiments on Lunatics," ibid., p. 842.

89. See Henry J. Berkley, letter to the editor, *Br. Med. J.*, 1897, *2*, 1297. Also see Berkley's letter to *Life*, 6 Dec. 1900, and the skeptical response, in "Dr. Berkley's Experiments," *J. Zoophily*, 1901, *10*, 18–20; and in *New England Anti-Vivisection Society Monthly*, Feb. 1901, 18–21.

90. W. H. Welch to W. W. Keen, 13 Dec. 1900; Sanarelli's original paper appeared in *Annali d'Igiene Sperimentale*, 1897, *7*, 441–49; *Sanarelli*, three-page handwritten memorandum, Keen Papers, CPP.

91. W. H. Welch to W. W. Keen, 1 Jan. 1901, Keen Papers, CPP.

92. W. H. Welch to W. W. Keen, 13 Dec. 1900; for the bacteriological limbo of Sanarelli's pathogen, see Margaret H. Warner, "Hunting the Yellow Fever Germ: The Principle and Practice of Etiological Proof in Late Nineteenth Century America," *Bull. Hist. Med.*, 1985, *59*, 361–82.

93. K. Menge's original paper, "Ueber ein bacterienfeindliches Verhalten der Scheidensecrete Nichtschwangerer," appeared in *Dtsch. Med. Wochenschr.*, 1894, *20*, 907–10.

94. "Vivisection and Antivivisection," p. 373.

95. W. H. Welch to W. W. Keen, 22 Mar. 1901, Keen Papers, CPP.

96. J. B. R., "Human Vivisection," *Philadelphia Polyclinic*, 1896, *5*, 357–58.

97. The Wentworth incident is described in Benison et al., *Walter B. Cannon*, pp. 176–78.

98. *The Reality of Human Vivisection*, p. 19.

99. Ibid.

100. Ibid., p. 31.

101. *Shall Science Do Murder?* (Philadelphia: American Anti-Vivisection Society, n.d.), p. 3, Antivivisection files, 600–1; box 2, f. 23, RUA.

102. "A Bill for the Regulation of Scientific Experiments upon Human Beings in the District of Columbia," S. 3424, 56th Cong., 1st sess., 2 Mar. 1900. The text of the bill appears in Appendix I of this volume.

103. "Experiments on Human Beings," *JAMA*, 1900, *34*, 696.

104. William W. Keen to Senator Gallinger, 21 Mar. 1900, Keen Papers, CPP.

Chapter Four

1. Walter Bradford Cannon, "The Responsibility of the General Practitioner for Freedom of Medical Research," *Boston Med. Surg. J.*, 1909, *161*, 430.

2. Saul Benison, A. Clifford Barger, and Elin L. Wolfe, *Walter B. Cannon* (Cambridge: Harvard University Press, 1987), p. 191.

3. Henry K. Beecher, *Research and the Individual* (Boston: Little, Brown, 1970), p. 221; and Donald E. Konold, *A History of American Medical Ethics* (Madison: State Historical Society of Wisconsin, 1962).

4. Sydney R. Taber, "Shall Vivisection Be Restricted?" letter to the editor of *Chicago Record-Herald*, 12 May 1905; and *Reasonable Restriction vs. Absolute License in Vivisection* (Chicago: Vivisection Reform Society, 1907).

5. Taber, "Shall Vivisection Be Restricted?"

6. S. R. Taber, *Illustrations of Human Vivisection* (Chicago: Vivisection Reform Society, 1906), p. 12; Mary C. Putnam, "On Atropine," *Med. Rec.*, 1873, *8*, 249–54; Mary Putnam Jacobi, "Sphygmographic Experiments upon a Human Brain Exposed by an Opening in the Cranium," *Am. J. Med. Sci.*, 1878, *76*, 10.

7. S. Weir Mitchell, W. W. Keen, and George R. Morehouse, "On the Antagonism of Atrophia and Morphia, Founded upon Observations and Experiments made at the U. S. A. Hospital for Injuries and Diseases of the Nervous System," *Am. J. Med. Sci.*, 1865, *50*, 71.

8. Keen defended the therapeutic intent of the studies; see William W. Keen, *Animal Experimentation and Medical Progress* (Boston: Houghton Mifflin, 1914), p. 236. Taber, *Illustrations of Human Vivisection*, p. 14.

9. Paul C. Freer, "Accidental Inoculation with the Virus of Plague," *JAMA*, 1907, *48*, 1264–65.

10. Eli Chernin, "Richard Pearson Strong and the Iatrogenic Plague Disaster in Bilibid Prison, Manila, 1906," *Rev. Infect. Dis.*, 1989, *11*, 1000.

11. S. R. Taber, "Recent Scientific Experimentation on Human Material," *J. Zoophily*, 1907, *16*, 94; and "Scientific Experimentation at Manila," *New York Evening Post*, 22 May 1907.

12. "Scientific Experimentation at Manila."

13. Joseph W. Stickler, "Foot-and-Mouth Disease as it Affects Man and Animals," *NY Med. J.*, 1887, *32*, 725–32. Also see his reports in *Med. Rec.*, 1887, *32*, 745–46, and *Boston Med. Surg. J.*, 1887, *117*, 607–9.

14. "A More Excellent Way of Scientific Research," *J. Zoophily*, 1906, *15*, 117.

15. See Harvey A. Levenstein, *Revolution at the Table* (New York: Oxford University Press, 1988), p. 90.

16. See "Rockefeller Institute Buys a Farm for Vivisection Plant," *New York Herald*, 20 Oct. 1907; "A Vivisection Farm," *New York Times*, 22 Oct. 1907.

17. Discussions of the fire appeared in the *New York Herald* and the *New York Globe*, 27 Nov. 1909 (in Newspaper Clipping Book, Antivivisection Files, RUA).

18. See "Origin of the *New York Herald*'s Antivivisection Propaganda," typescript prepared by Fred W. Eastman (assistant to Frederic Schiller Lee, professor of physiology at Columbia University), 19 June 1911, Antivivisection Files, RUA.

19. "Mrs. Eames Aids Vivisection Fight," *New York Herald*, 12 Feb. 1908.

20. See *New York Herald*, 27 Dec. 1909; Flexner's reply in *New York Times*, 17 Jan. 1910; "Defense of Medical Research," *JAMA*, 1910, *54*, 477, reports Mary Kennedy's case against the Rockefeller Institute.

21. George W. Corner, *A History of the Rockefeller Institute 1901–1953* (New York: Rockefeller Institute Press, 1964), pp. 85–86.

22. See editorials in *New York Times*, 24 Feb. and 26 Feb. 1908; editorial in *New York Evening Post*, 5 Mar. 1908; and the editorial in *NY Med. J.*, 1908, *87*, 29–30. For the retraction see ibid., p. 73.

23. William J. Shultz, *The Humane Movement in the United States, 1910–1922* (1924; New York: AMS Press, 1968), pp. 153–56.

24. Diana Belais, "Vivisection Animal and Human," *Cosmopolitan*, 1910, *50*, 267–73; for Hearst's reorientation of the magazine, see Frank Luther Mott, *A History of American Magazines 1885–1905* (Cambridge: Harvard University Press, 1957), pp. 494–97.

25. Samuel McClintock Hamill, Howard C. Carpenter, and Thomas A. Cope, "A Comparison of the von Pirquet, Calmette, and Moro Tuberculin Tests and Their Diagnostic Value," *Arch. Int. Med.*, 1908, *2*, 405. For clinical investigation in Philadelphia, see A. McGehee Harvey, *Science at the Bedside: Clinical Research in American Medicine, 1905–1945* (Baltimore: Johns Hopkins University Press, 1981), pp. 206–11.

26. Quoted in *Tuberculin Tests on Human Beings* (Philadelphia: American Anti-Vivisection Society, n.d.), p. 3.

27. Belais, "Vivisection Animal and Human," pp. 270–71.

28. See Susan E. Lederer, "Orphans as Guinea Pigs: American Children and Medical Experimenters, 1890–1930," in *In the Name of the Child: Health and Social Policy, 1870–1940*, ed. Roger Cooter (London: Routledge, 1992), pp. 96–123.

29. Henderson challenged the physicians to attempt experiments on her "six, robust, unvaccinated and otherwise untampered-with children"; see Jessica C. Henderson, "Antivivisection," *J. Zoophily*, 1913, *22*, 45.

30. L. Emmett Holt, "A Report on One Thousand Tuberculin Tests in Young Children," *Arch. Pediatr.*, 1909, *26*, 1. R. L. Duffus and L. Emmett Holt, Jr., *L. Emmett Holt, Pioneer of a Children's Century* (New York: D. Appleton, 1940), pp. 164–65.

31. Diana Belais, *Vivisection—A Menace to Hospital Patients* (New York: Vivisection Investigation League, n.d.), p. 3.

32. Louis Hamman and Samuel Wolman, "The Cutaneous and Conjunctival Tuberculin Tests in the Diagnosis of Pulmonary Tuberculosis," *Arch. Int. Med.*, 1909, *3*, 307–49.

33. *Tuberculin Tests on Human Beings* (New York: Vivisection Investigation League, n.d.).

34. W. H. Wilder, "Report of the Committee for the Study of the Relation of Tuberculosis to Diseases of the Eye," *JAMA*, 1910, *55*, 21–24.

35. Hideyo Noguchi, "A Cutaneous Reaction in Syphilis," *J. Exp. Med.*, 1911, *14*, 557–68. See also Susan E. Lederer, "Hideyo Noguchi's Luetin Experiment and the Antivivisectionists," *Isis*, 1985, *76*, 31–48.

36. See Corner, *A History of the Rockefeller Institute*, pp. 84–87; and Harry F. Dowling, *Fighting Infection Conquests of the Twentieth Century* (Cambridge: Harvard University Press, 1977), pp. 84–94.

37. Hideyo Noguchi, "Experimental Research in Syphilis with Especial Reference to *Spirochaeta pallida (Treponema pallidum)*," *JAMA*, 1912, *68*, 1163–72.

38. Noguchi explained that the word *normal* meant free of syphilis; Hideyo Noguchi to William Williams Keen, 21 Nov. 1912, Keen Papers, CPP.

39. Jerome D. Green to Charles S. Whitman, 16 May 1912, Faculty-Noguchi Correspondence, RUA.

40. Correspondence of Henry James, Jr., with legal firm of Fish, Richardson, Herrick and Neave, 1913–14, Business Manager's Files, RUA.

41. *Human Vivisection* (New York Anti-Vivisection Society, n. d.); *What Vivisection Inevitably Leads To* (Vivisection Investigation League, n. d.).

42. Henderson, "Antivivisection," p. 45.

43. Allan M. Brandt, *No Magic Bullet: A Social History of Venereal Disease in the United States since 1880* (Oxford: Oxford University Press, 1985) discusses the rise of the social hygiene movement and changes in attitudes toward venereal infection in the twentieth century.

44. See John C. Burnham, "The Progressive Era Revolution in American Attitudes toward Sex," *J. Am. Hist.*, 1973, *59*, 885–908.

45. J. W. Churchman, *The Value of Animal Experimentation as Illustrated by Recent Advances in the Study of Syphilis, Defense of Research Pamphlet XX* (Chicago: American Medical Association, 1911).

46. C. E. White to W. W. Keen, 14 May 1911, Keen Papers, CPP.

47. W. W. Keen to C. E. White, 18 May 1911, Keen Papers, CPP.

48. See John Ettling, *The Germ of Laziness: Rockefeller Philanthropy and Public Health in the New South* (Cambridge: Harvard University Press, 1981), pp. 184–85.

49. "The Only Explanation," *Life*, 1909, *54*, 68.

50. This release appeared 18 October 1910 in the following New York newspapers: *American, Evening Telegram, Herald, Times*, and *Sun* (Newspaper Clipping Book, Antivivisection Files, RUA). For charges of brutality at New York hospitals, see "Physicians Ridicule Barnesby's Charges," *New York Times*, 1 Nov. 1910.

51. Corner, *A History of the Rockefeller Institute*, pp. 96–97.

52. Frank Stephens, "The Existing Evidence of Experiments on Human Beings," in *Proceedings of the International Anti-Vivisection and Animal Protection Congress Held at Washington, D.C., December 8th to 11th, 1913* (New York: Tudor Press, [1914?]), p. 95.

53. See, for example, "The Inevitable Tendency of Vivisection," *J. Zoophily*, 1913, *22*, 398.

54. "Too Much Courtesy," *Life*, 1912, *60*, 2495.

55. This language is discussed in Ross G. Mitchell, "The Child and Experimental Medicine," *Br. Med. J.*, 1964, *1*, 721–27. For Holt's "professional etiquette," see *Vivisection—A Menace to Hospital Patients*.

56. Jerome D. Greene, "Note," Antivivisection Files, RUA; this one-page statement was approved by Noguchi 19 June 1912. See Greene to Walter B. Cannon, 21 June 1912, RUA, RG 199.11.

57. See Isabel R. Plesset, *Noguchi and His Patrons* (Rutherford, N.J.: Fairleigh Dickinson University Press, 1980), pp. 146–48.

58. Jerome D. Greene to District Attorney Charles S. Whitman, 16 May 1912, Faculty-Noguchi Correspondence, RUA.

59. Jerome D. Greene to Starr J. Murphy, 22 May 1912, Board of Trustees—Counsel Correspondence, RUA.

60. See "Baseless Charge Against Dr. Noguchi," *New York Times*, 21 May 1912; "This Outrage Should Be Punished," ibid., 22 May 1912; "Unintentional Murderers," *New York Globe*, 21 May 1912; and "Piling Up Slander on Slander," *New York Times*, 10 June 1912.

61. *The Bill to Prohibit Human Vivisection (Abstract from Pennsylvania Legislative Journals of April 16th and 29th, 1913, of Argument of Hon. Henry E. Lanius in support of House Bill 1225 To Prohibit Experiment on Human Beings)*, pamphlet, (n.p., n.d.), RUA, RG 600-1, box 2, f. 23. See also "Human Vivisection," *American Anti-Vivisection Society 30th Annual Report* (Philadelphia, 1913), pp. 38–45.

62. Henry E. Lanius, "The Danger of Experimenting on Human Beings," *Proceedings of the International Anti-Vivisection and Animal Protection Congress*, pp. 166–70.

63. John B. Blake, "The Inoculation Controversy in Boston, 1721–1722," in

Sickness and Health in America, ed. Judith Walzer Leavitt and Ronald L. Numbers (Madison: University of Wisconsin Press, 1985), pp. 347–55.

64. Stephens, "The Existing Evidence," p. 97. Karl von Ruck, "A Practical Method of Prophylactic Immunization against Tuberculosis," *Med. Rec.*, 1912, *82*, 369–80, at p. 371.

65. "Government to Test Von Ruck's Vaccine," *New York Tribune*, 30 Mar. 1913, p. 20; "Dr. Von Ruck's Tuberculin, *New York Times*, 26 June 1913, p. 8; and "Split on Von Ruck Tests," *New York Times*, 20 Oct. 1913.

66. See "Wilson Opposed to Vivisection," *New York Times*, 10 Dec. 1913, p. 11. Also see "Professional Libellers," *Columbus Dispatch* (Ohio), 13 Dec. 1913; "Children Prey of Vivisectors, Say Delegates," *New York American*, 9 Dec. 1913; "Denies Charge of Human Vivisection," *Baltimore Evening News*, 11 Dec. 1913; and "Vivisection Foes Meet," *New York Times*, 9 Dec. 1913.

67. Karl von Ruck to W. W. Keen, 13 Dec. 1913, Keen Papers, CPP.

68. A. M. Stimson, "Report on the Investigations of the Methods and Practices Employed by Drs. Karl and Silvio von Ruck in Treating Tuberculosis and in Rendering Persons Immune from Tuberculosis," in *Treatment of Tuberculosis* Senate doc. 641, 63rd Cong., 3rd sess., (Washington, D.C.: Government Printing Office, 1914), p. 5.

69. Stephens, "The Existing Evidence," 96–97. For the ringworm study, see F. C. Knowles, "Molluscum Contagiosum: Report of An Institutional Epidemic of Fifty-nine Cases," *JAMA*, 1909, *53*, 671–73. Also see *The Rise and Fall of A Vaccine With the Indiscriminate Use of Children and Animals* (New York: Vivisection Investigation League, n.d.).

70. "Experimenting on Insane," *Med. Rec.*, 1913, *83*, 583; Henry James, Jr., to Senator G. A. Blauvelt, 25 Feb. 1914. Senator Herrick introduced an earlier version of the bill 11 Mar. 1913; see RUA, RG 600–1, box 1, f. 10. The New Jersey legislature's Committee on Public Health reviewed Assembly bill no. 486, introduced 25 Feb. 1914.

71. See the following stories in the *New York American*: "U.S. Senate to Inquire into Vivisection In N.Y.," 17 Feb. 1914; "Babies, Blood, and Science," 16 Feb. 1914; "Dual Probe of Child Infection Begins Today," 20 Feb. 1914; "Experiments on 1,000 Babies," and "Hideyo Noguchi," 14 Feb. 1914; "Children Suffered Under Test, Says Mrs. Farrell," 16 Feb. 1914; "Flexner's Japanese Aid Describes Serum Method," 15 Feb. 1914; "Vivisection of Infants Subject of City Inquiry," 16 Feb. 1914; "Flexner Defends Human Vivisection," 15 Feb. 1914; and "Inoculation of Fifty-Two Children to Go to Bronx Grand Jury," 18 Feb. 1914.

72. "Boy with Nasal Illness Inoculated in the Arm, Dies," *New York American*, 19 Feb. 1914; "Child's Measles 'Doctored' into Dread Disease," *New York American*, 17 Feb. 1914; and "Father Sues Hospital over Experiment on His Child," *New York Times*, 11 May 1913.

73. "Absurd Charges Refuted," *Weekly Bulletin of the New York City Department of Health*, 28 Feb. 1914, n.s. *3*, 1–2.

74. Sigismund S. Goldwater, Commissioner of Health, to William H. Maxwell, New York City Superintendent of Schools, 27 Feb. 1914, RUA, RG 600–1, box 1, f. 11.

75. Katharine Loving Buell, "A Campaign of Lies," *Harper's Weekly*, 16 May 1914, *58*, 15. See also "Another Antivivisection Fiasco," *JAMA*, 1914, *62*, 1025; "Vivisection Again," *Long Isl. Med. J.*, 1914, *8*, 103–4.

76. "Questionnaire," New York Anti-Vivisection Society, Antivivisection Files, RUA. For one physician's response, see F. H. Todd, M.D., "A Medical Opinion on Vivisection," *Open Door*, Mar. 1916, p. 6.

77. "Minutes of the Board of Scientific Directors and Executive Committee," 7 Jan. 1914, RUA. For successful libel suits, see "A Righteous Verdict Against an Antivivisectionist," *JAMA*, 1903, *41*, 1305; "An Antivivisection Leader," *JAMA*, 1910, *54*, 540; and "A Year in Prison for Libelling Ehrlich," *Am. Med.*, 1914, *20*, 389–90.

78. James B. Reynolds to Henry James, Jr., 18 Dec. 1913, RUA, RG 600–1, box 1, f. 10.

79. Jerome D. Greene to Starr J. Murphy, 14 May 1912, Board of Trustees—Counsel Correspondence, RUA.

80. Jerome D. Greene to Mrs. C. P. Farrell, 10 June 1912, RUA, RG 600–1, box 5, f. 12.

81. Henry James, Jr., to Walter B. Cannon, 26 Feb. 1914, RUA, RG 600–1, box 6, f. 2.

82. Henry James, Jr., to Starr J. Murphy, 19 Dec. 1913, Board of Trustees—Counsel Correspondence, RUA.

83. For Cohen, see *Experiments on Human Beings Continue* (New York: Vivisection Investigation League, n.d.).

84. Henry James, Jr., to H. K. Mulford Co., 9 and 10 July 1914, RUA, Business Manager's Files, RG 210.1.

85. Richard M. Pearce, *The Charge of "Human Vivisection" As Presented in Antivivisection Literature* (Chicago: American Medical Association, 1914), p. 3.

86. R. M. Pearce to Simon Flexner, 26 Feb. 1914, RUA, RG 600–1, box 6, f. 7. See George W. Corner, *Two Centuries of Medicine* (Philadelphia: J. B. Lippincott, 1965), pp. 242–44.

87. J. W. Stickler, "Foot-and-Mouth Disease as it Affects Man and Animals," *NY Med. J.*, 1887, *32*, 725–32; see Pearce, *Charge of "Human Vivisection,"* p. 6. The accounts of Stickler's death differ as to the date and cause: "Necrology," *JAMA*, 1899, *32*, 1269; Henry Heiman, "Obituary of Joseph Stickler (1854–1899)," *Trans. Med. Soc. NJ*, 1899, 286–88.

88. Pearce, *Charge of "Human Vivisection,"* p. 24.

89. M. J. Rodermund, "Medical Wonders and Medical Blunders—A Story of Facts," *Medical Brief*, 1906, *34*, 279–83, on p. 282. For a letter to *Life* disputing Rodermund's status as a "true scientist," see "From a Physician," *Life*, 1910, *55*, 949. See also *Vivisectors Clamor for Human Beings to Vivisect* (New York: New York Anti-Vivisection Society, n.d.).

90. Pearce, *Charge of "Human Vivisection,"* pp. 24–25.

91. Joseph Erlanger to Walter B. Cannon, 3 May 1909, Cannon Papers, HMS. See also M. J. Rodermund to Joseph Erlanger, 12 Feb. 1910, Cannon Papers, HMS. Also see Benison et al., *Walter B. Cannon*, pp. 274–76.

92. J. L. Yates to Walter B. Cannon, 11 May 1909; Yates to Cannon, 12 July 1910; clipping from *Milwaukee Journal*, 12 July 1910, Cannon Papers, HMS.

93. Pearce, *Charge of "Human Vivisection,"* p. 30.

94. Richard M. Pearce to Walter B. Cannon, 27 Mar. 1914, Cannon Papers, HMS.

95. "A Caution to Medical Writers," *JAMA*, 1901, *37*, 1120.

96. George B. Broad, "Laboratory Aid in Surgical Technique," *Med. Rec.*, 1901, *60*, 615–16.

97. The advertisement for Lederle vaccine appeared in the *Am. J. Pub. Health*, Feb. 1914; see W. B. Cannon to Henry James, 19 Oct. 1914, and James to Cannon, 21 Oct. 1914, RUA, RG 600–1, box 6, f. 2.

98. "The Pathogenicity of Amebas," *JAMA*, 1914, *62*, 300–301. Keen may not have read the editorial closely; it did describe the subjects as volunteers (see W. W. Keen to Henry James, Jr., 27 Jan. 1914, RUA, RG 600–1).

99. "Report of the Committee on the Protection of Medical Research," *JAMA*, 1914, *63*, 94.

100. "Protecting Medical Research," *Chicago Med. Rec.*, 1914, *36*, 360; see replies to Cannon's circular from editors of *J. Abnormal Psych.*, *Am. J. Insanity*, *Southwest J. Med. Surg.*, May 1914, Cannon Papers, HMS.

101. Udo J. Wile, "Experimental Syphilis in the Rabbit Produced by the Brain Substance of the Living Paretic," *J. Exp. Med.*, 1916, *23*, 199–202. See also Susan E. Lederer, "'The Right and Wrong of Making Experiments on Human Beings': Udo J. Wile and Syphilis," *Bull. Hist. Med.*, 1984, *58*, 380–97.

102. For Wile's life, see obituary, *New York Times*, 8 June 1965; Arthur C. Curtis and Edward P. Cawley, "Tribute to Dr. Udo J. Wile," *Arch. Dermat. Syphil.*, 1949, *60*, 139–42.

103. Udo J. Wile, "The Demonstration of the *Spirochaeta pallida* in the Brain Substance of Living Paretics (Forster and Tomaszczewski)," *JAMA*, 1913, *61*, 866.

104. See Hideyo Noguchi, "The Transmission of *Treponema pallidum* from the Brains of Paretics to the Rabbit," *JAMA*, 1913, *61*, 85; Henry J. Nichols, "Observations on a Strain of *Spirochaeta pallida* Isolated from the Nervous System," *J. Exp. Med.*, 1914, *19*, 362–71; and John A. F. Pfeiffer, "A Note Concerning Strains of *Treponema pallidum* Obtained from the Brains of Paretics at Autopsy," *Proc. Soc. Exp. Biol. Med.*, 1916–17, *14*, 1–3.

105. For information on the Pontiac State Hospital, see Colonel B. Burr, *Medical History of Michigan*, 2 vols., (St. Paul, Minn.: Bruce Publishing, 1930).

106. Wile, "Demonstration of the *Spirochaeta*," p. 866.

107. *Human Beings Vivisected* (New York: Vivisection Investigation League, 1916).

108. Ibid., p. 4.

109. See "Human Vivisection Arouses Protest," *New York Herald*, 12 Apr. 1916; "Silly Uproar," *Detroit News*, 13 Apr. 1916; and "Experiments on Insane Humans," *Detroit News*, 14 Apr. 1916.

110. "Human Vivisection," *Living Tissue*, 1916, *1*, 2–3; see "Human Vivisection," *Philadelphia Inquirer*, 14 Apr. 1916.

111. "Vivisection on Human Beings," *Chicago Daily Tribune*, 12 Apr. 1916.

112. Quoted in "Human Vivisection—the Betrayal of a Sacred Trust," *Our Dumb Animals*, 1916, *49*, 34.

113. Simon Flexner to William Williams Keen, 19 Apr. 1916, W. W. Keen Papers, APS.

114. Henry James, Jr., to Walter Bradford Cannon, 24 Apr. 1916, Antivivisection Files, RUA.

115. Walter B. Cannon to Simon Flexner, 7 June 1916, Simon Flexner Papers, APS; Cannon to Henry James, Jr., 25 Apr. 1916, Antivivisection Files, RUA.

116. Copy of letter sent to Udo J. Wile also sent to Victor C. Vaughan, 27 Apr. 1916, Victor C. Vaughan Papers, MHC.

117. Walter B. Cannon to F. S. Lee, 12 May 1916, F. S. Lee Papers, CPS, box 1, f. 25.

118. Henry James, Jr., to Walter B. Cannon, 24 Apr. 1916, Antivivisection Files, RUA.

119. Simon Flexner to Walter B. Cannon, 6 June 1916, Simon Flexner Papers, APS.

120. Rufus Cole to Francis Peabody, 1 June 1916, Rufus Cole Papers, APS.

121. Ibid.

122. Francis Peabody to Walter B. Cannon, 19 May 1916, F. S. Lee Papers, CPS, box 1, f. 25.

123. Ibid.

124. William Williams Keen to Henry James, Jr., 29 Apr. 1916, Antivivisection Files, RUA; Keen to Victor C. Vaughan, 15 June 1916, Vaughan Papers, MHC.

125. W. W. Keen, "The Inveracities of Antivivisection," *JAMA*, 1916, *67*, 1390–91. William Williams Keen to Victor C. Vaughan, 15 June 1916; and Vaughan to Keen, 25 Apr. 1916, Victor C. Vaughan Papers, MHC.

126. [W. B. Cannon], "The Right and Wrong of Making Experiments on Human Beings," *JAMA*, 1916, *67*, 1372–73.

127. Cannon, "The Right and Wrong," p. 1373.

Chapter Five

1. *Your Baby and Your Dog* (New York: Vivisection Investigation League, n.d.).

2. Albert T. Leffingwell, *An Ethical Problem; or, Sidelights upon Scientific Experimentation on Man and Animals,* 2nd ed., rev. (New York: C. P. Farrell, 1916), p. 324.

3. Walter B. Cannon to Richard M. Pearce, 9 Jan. 1915, Cannon Papers, HMS.

4. See "Anti-Vivisection U.S. Senators," *J. Zoophily*, 1918, *26*, 154.

5. William W. Keen, "The Red Cross and the Antivivisectionists," *Science*, 1918, *47*, 175–82; "Antivivisectionists Attack the Red Cross," *JAMA*, 1919, *72*, 280; and "Antivivisectionists Seek to Cripple Nation's Defense," *JAMA*, 1922, *79*, 1521–23.

6. Cornelia James Cannon, "Is the Woman Vote Sentimental?" *Woman Citizen*, 30 Dec. 1922, p. 16.

7. Simon Flexner and James Thomas Flexner, *William Henry Welch and the Heroic Age of American Medicine* (New York: The Viking Press, 1941), p. 262.

8. "Fifty Years Young," *The A-V*, 1945, *53*, 33.

9. Susan E. Lederer, "Political Animals: The Shaping of Biomedical Research Literature in Twentieth-Century America," *Isis*, 1992, *83*, 61–79.

10. Charles Hermann, "Immunization Against Measles," *Arch. Pediatr.*, 1915, *32*, 506.

11. Claud D. Johnson and Ernest W. Goodpasture, "The Etiology of Mumps," *Am. J. Hygiene*, 1935, *21*, 47.

12. Susan E. Lederer and Michael A. Grodin, "Historical Overview: Pediatric Experimentation," in *Children as Research Subjects: Science, Ethics, and Law*, ed. Michael A. Grodin and Leonard Glantz (New York: Oxford University Press, 1994), pp. 3–25.

13. Agnes F. Chase, "The Modern Moloch," *The A-V*, 1943, *51*, 9. See also Paul de Kruif, "We Can Wipe Out Whooping Cough," *Reader's Digest*, 1943, 125.

14. H. MacDonald and E. J. MacDonald, "Experimental Pertussis," *J. Inf. Dis.*, 1933, *53*, 328–30. For a pediatrician who similarly challenged a measles vaccine by "painting" the throats of immunized infants with nasal secretions of patients with active measles, see Katsuji Kato, "The Bacteriology and Serotherapy of Measles," *Am. J. Dis. Child.*, 1928, *36*, 536.

15. Leon Goldman, "History of Self-Experimentation in Dermatology: Should We Go First—Sometimes?" *Cutis*, 1991, *48*, 338–41.

16. "Heard and Read," *The Starry Cross*, 1933, *41*, 34. See T. Toyoda, Y. Futagi, and M. Okamoto, "Experimental Production of Scarlet Fever by Means of a Scarlatinal Hemolytic Streptococcus," *J. Infect. Dis.*, 1931, *48*, 350–57.

17. Alfred F. Hess and Mildred Fish, "Infantile Scurvy: The Blood, the Blood-Vessels, and the Diet," *Am. J. Dis. Child.*, 1914, *8*, 386–405.

18. Konrad Bercovici, "Orphans as Guinea Pigs," *The Nation*, 1921, *112*, 913.

19. "Orphans and Dietetics," *Am. Med.*, 1921, *27*, 394–96.

20. M. Hines Roberts, "The Spinal Fluid in the New-Born," *JAMA*, 1925, *85*, 500.

21. Ibid., p. 501.

22. "Heard and Read," *The Starry Cross*, 1928, *37*, 59.

23. "Monkey Shines," *The Starry Cross*, 1934, *42*, 124.

24. John A. Kolmer, George F. Klugh, Jr., and Anna M. Rule, "A Successful Method for Vaccination Against Acute Anterior Poliomyelitis," *JAMA*, 1935, *104*, 456–60.

25. From April to September, 1935, 10,725 children received the Kolmer vaccine. Brodie's field tests included 9,000 vaccinated children and 4,500 controls. Lawrence B. Berk, "Polio Vaccine Trials of 1935," *Trans. Stud. Coll. Physicians Phila.*, 1989, *11*, 321–26; and Maurice Brodie and William H. Park, "Active Immunization Against Poliomyelitis," *JAMA*, 1935, *105*, 1089–93.

26. See "Trial of Physicians Following the Lubeck Disaster," *JAMA*, 1931, *97*, 403.

27. John R. Paul, *A History of Poliomyelitis* (New Haven: Yale University Press, 1971), pp. 252–62.

28. "Equal Rights for Orphans," *National Humane Review*, Feb. 1934, p. 14.

29. Naomi Rogers, *Dirt and Disease: Polio before FDR* (New Brunswick, N.J.: Rutgers University Press, 1992), pp. 165–71.

30. John A. Kolmer to E. C. Williams, 15 Oct. 1934, United States Public Health Service General Files, RG 90, National Archives. I am grateful to Sydney Halpern for this reference.

31. William H. Park to E. C. Williams, 17 Oct. 1934, U.S. Public Health Service, RG 90, National Archives.

32. "Paralysis Serum Not For Babies Yet," *New York Times*, 27 Apr. 1932.

33. F. P. Rous to Walter B. Cannon, 1 June 1932, RUA, RG 600–1, box 17, f. 12.

34. F. Peyton Rous to William C. Black, 21 July 1941, F. P. Rous Papers, APS, f. JEM-Black. Rous's editorial policies are discussed in Lederer, "Political Animals," pp. 61–79.

35. William C. Black, "The Etiology of Acute Infectious Gingivostomatitis (Vincent's Stomatitis)," *J. Pediatr.*, 1942, *30*, 153.

36. Elizabeth Etheridge, *The Butterfly Caste: A Social History of Pellagra* (Westport, Conn.: Greenwood, 1972), pp. 93–96.

37. Ernest Linwood Walker and Andrew Watson Sellards, "Experimental Entamoebic Dysentery," *Phil. J. Sci.*, 1913, *8*, 259.

38. Ibid., p. 323.

39. Richard P. Strong and B. C. Crowell, "Etiology of Beriberi," *Phil. J. Sci.*, 1912, *7*, 271–414.

40. Quoted in Etheridge, *The Butterfly Caste*, p. 95.

41. Jon M. Harkness discusses research on prisoners in "Inmates and Experiments: A History of Nontherapeutic Medical Research" (Ph.D. diss., University of Wisconsin, in progress).

42. "A Recent Case of Human Experimentation," *Open Door*, Nov. 1915, p. 4.

43. L. L. Stanley, "Experiences in Testicle Transplantation," *Calif. St. J. Med.*, 1920, *18*, 251–53.

44. *Before the Bar of Public Opinion* (California Anti-Vivisection Society, n.d.), Hooper Papers, AR 59–1 f. 76, UCSF.

45. "Crooks for Vivisection," *J. Zoophily*, 1917, *26*, 41.

46. Robert Logan, "Criminal Guinea Pigs," *The Starry Cross*, 1935, *43*, 19.

47. For France: "Human Vivisection," *The Abolitionist*, 1 Nov. 1927, p. 157; for England: "A Use for Condemned Murderers," *JAMA*, 1929, *92*, 67; for Mexico: F. Castillo Najera, "La Experimentación en los séres humanos ante nuestra Ley Penal," *Gac. Med. Mex.*, 1923, *55*, 747–51.

48. Logan, "Criminal Guinea Pigs," p. 19.

49. "Tuberculosis Test Reported Success," *New York Times*, 11 Dec. 1934.

50. Charles E. Simon, *Human Infection Carriers* (Philadelphia: Lea & Febiger, 1919), p. 101.

51. H. J. Nichols, J. S. Simmons, and C. O. Stimmel, "The Surgical Treatment of Typhoid Carriers," *JAMA*, 1919, *73*, 680. On courts-martial for refusing a surgical operation, see W. H. Johnson, "Civil Rights of Military Personnel Regarding Medical Care and Experimental Procedures," *Science*, 1953, *117*, 212–15.

52. William S. Dow, "The Possibility of Medical Research in the Military Service Because of Its Complete Control Over Personnel," *Mil. Surg.*, 1925, *56*, 131.

53. "Statement of George Martin Kober," in *A Vindication of Vivisection: A Course of Lectures on Animal Experimentation,* ed. Francis A. Tondorf (Washington, D.C., 1920), p. 375. See also chapter 6 in this volume.

54. Susan E. Lederer, "Experimentation on Military Personnel," in *Encyclopedia of Bioethics* (New York: Macmillan, forthcoming).

55. W. D. Tigertt, "The Initial Effort to Immunize American Soldier Volunteers with Typhoid Vaccine," *Mil. Med.,* 1959, *124,* 342–49.

56. Charles F. Kieffer, "Smokeless Powders," *JAMA,* 1905, *44,* 1359–65.

57. James S. Stevens and Joe H. St. John, and Francois H. K. Reynolds, "Experimental Studies of Dengue," *Phil. J. Sci.,* 1931, *44,* 162.

58. Leffingwell, *An Ethical Problem,* p. 320.

59. See Donald G. Bates, "The Background to John Young's Thesis on Digestion," *Bull. Hist. Med.,* 1962, *36,* 341–61, for an antebellum physician's use of a subject, who earned his livelihood swallowing stones in a traveling troupe, to study digestion.

60. Ronald L. Numbers, "William Beaumont and the Ethics of Human Experimentation," *J. Hist. Biol.,* 1979, *12,* 117.

61. Edward C. Atwater, "'Squeezing Mother Nature': Experimental Physiology in the United States before 1870," *Bull. Hist. Med.,* 1978, *52,* 314.

62. René Fülöp-Miller, *Triumph Over Pain* (Indianapolis: Bobbs-Merrill, 1938), p. 123.

63. J. Marion Sims, *The Story of My Life* (New York: D. Appleton, 1894), p. 236.

64. Ibid., p. 246.

65. Todd L. Savitt, "The Use of Blacks for Medical Experimentation and Demonstration in the Old South," *J. South. Hist.,* 1982, *48,* 331–48.

66. Emanuel Snydacker, "Trachoma," *JAMA,* 1899, *32,* 213.

67. C. A. Herter to Ira Remsen, 26 Feb. 1910, Remsen Papers, Johns Hopkins University; and James Harvey Young, "Saccharin: A Bitter Regulatory Controversy," in *Research in the Administration of Public Policy,* ed. Frank B. Evans and Harold T. Pinkett (Washington, D.C.: Howard University Press, 1975), pp. 32–49.

68. Ludy T. Benjamin, Jr., Anne M. Rogers, and Angela Rosenbaum, "Coca-Cola, Caffeine, and Mental Deficiency: Harry Hollingworth and the Chattanooga Trial of 1911," *J. Hist. Behav. Sci.,* 1991, *27,* 42–55.

69. "The Influence of Caffein on Mental and Motor Efficiency and on the Circulation," *JAMA,* 1912, *58,* 784–85; and Harry Hollingworth, "The Influence of Caffein on Mental and Motor Efficiency," *Arch. Psychol.,* 1912, *22,* 6–15.

70. Edward Reynolds and Robert W. Lovett, "An Experimental Study of Certain Phases of Chronic Backache," *JAMA,* 1910, *54,* 1036. For another use of an artist's model, see Francis G. Benedict, "A Photographic Method for Measuring the Surface Area of the Human Body," *Am. J. Phys.,* 1916, *41,* 275–91.

71. Asa C. Chandler and Lee Rice, "Observations on the Etiology of Dengue Fever," *Am. J. Trop. Med.,* 1923, *3,* 255.

72. See Olaf Bergeim, John M. Evvard, Martin E. Rehfuss and Philip B. Hawk, "A

Fractional Study of the Coagulation of Milk in the Human Stomach," *Am. J. Phys.*, 1919, *48*, 411–18.

73. R. S. Lavenson, "Observations on a Child With a Gastric Fistula in Relation to Recent Advances in the Physiology of Gastric Digestion," *Arch. Intern. Med.*, 1909, *4*, 271–90.

74. Anton Julius Carlson, *The Control of Hunger in Health and Disease* (Chicago: University of Chicago Press, 1916), p. 30.

75. A. J. Carlson, "The Character of the Movements of the Empty Stomach in Man," *Am. J. Phys.*, 1912–13, *31*, 151.

76. Numbers, "William Beaumont," p. 132.

77. A. J. Carlson, "The Influence of the Gastric Mucosa on the Contractions of the Empty Stomach (Hunger Contractions) in Man," *Am. J. Phys.*, 1913, *32*, 251–52.

78. A. J. Carlson, "The Hunger Contractions of the Empty Stomach During Prolonged Starvation (Man, Dog)," *Am. J. Phys.*, 1914, *33*, 95–118.

79. For Benedict's difficulties with Levansin, see *New York Times*, 5 May 1912, p. 11; 15 May 1912, p. 10; 21 May 1912, p. 24; 22 May 1912, p. 11; and 27 May 1912, p. 4.

80. H. Ginsburg, I. Tumpowsky, and A. J. Carlson, "The Onset of Hunger in Infants After Feeding," *JAMA*, 1915, *64*, 1822–23. See Katharine S. Nicholson, "Anti-Vivisection Notes," *J. Zoophily*, 1917, *26*, 187–88.

81. Carlson, *The Control of Hunger*, p. 138.

82. Stewart Wolf and Harold G. Wolff, *Human Gastric Function: An Experimental Study of a Man and His Stomach* (New York: Oxford University Press, 1943), p. 98.

83. *Philadelphia Evening Bulletin* quoted in "Heard and Read," *The Starry Cross*, 1933, *41*, 59.

84. See N. S. Ferry, "Reappearance of Reaction at Site of Previous Dick Test Coincident with Appearance of Measles Rash in a Case of Measles," *JAMA*, 1926, *87*, 241–42; Janet Golden, "From Wet Nurse Directory to Milk Bank: The Delivery of Human Milk in Boston, 1909–1927," *Bull. Hist. Med.*, 1988, *62*, 589–605; and Charles V. Nemo, "I Sell Blood," *American Mercury*, 1934, *31*, 194–203.

85. M. Beddow Bayly, "Infantile Paralysis and Serum Treatment," *The Starry Cross*, 1935, *43*, 14.

86. For a male professional blood donor as research subject, see Fred W. Oberst and E. D. Plass, "Blood Changes Induced by Venesection in Women with Toxemia of Late Pregnancy," *J. Clin. Inv.*, 1940, *19*, 439–96. See "'Ghost' Fathers: Children Provided for the Childless," *News-week*, 12 May 1934, p. 16.

87. G. A. Talbert, "Changes in the Hydrogen Ion Concentration of the Urine, As A Result of Work and Heat," *Am. J. Phys.*, 1919, *50*, 580.

88. G. A. Talbert, "Effect of Work and Heat on the Hydrogen Ion Concentration of the Sweat," *Am. J. Phys.*, 1919, *50*, 439.

89. L. P. Herrington, "The Influence of Ionized Air Upon Normal Subjects," *J. Clin. Invest.*, 1935, *14*, 72.

90. Douglas P. Murphy, Rosemary Shoemaker, and Marion Rea, "Menstrual Re-

sponse to Luteinizing Extract of Pregnancy Urine," *Endocrinology*, 1934, *18*, 203–5.

91. "Offers Body and Life for Medical Tests," *New York Times*, 11 Dec. 1927. There was no report of researchers availing themselves of this offer.

92. William F. Petersen and Samuel A. Levinson, "General Correlations in One Hundred So-Called Normal Men," *Arch. Path.*, 1930, *9*, 151–82.

93. James H. Jones, *Bad Blood* (New York: Free Press, 1981).

94. Eunice Rivers, Stanley H. Schuman, Lloyd Simpson, and Sidney Olansky, "Twenty Years of Followup Experience In a Long-Range Medical Study," *Public Health Rep.*, 1953, *58*, 393.

95. Ibid., p. 394.

96. See Morton Mintz and Jerry S. Cohen, "Human Guinea Pigs," *Progressive*, 1976, *40*, 32–36; Jones, *Bad Blood*, pp. 216–19.

97. For William Osler Abbott (1902–1943), whose mother, Georgina Osler, was a niece of Sir William Osler, see William C. Stadie, "William Osler Abbott," *Trans. Assoc. Am. Physicians*, 1944, *58*, 7–9. For the intubation technique, see T. Grier Miller and W. Osler Abbott, "Intestinal Intubation: A Practical Technique," *Am. J. Med. Sci.*, 1934, *187*, 595–99.

98. W. Osler Abbott, "The Problem of the Professional Guinea Pig," *Proceedings of the Charaka Club*, 1941, *10*, 249–60.

99. Ibid., p. 253.

100. Ibid., p. 255.

101. Ibid., p. 259.

102. "Heard and Read," *The Starry Cross*, 1933, *41*, 59.

103. N. C. Williams, "Eighteen Women," *The A-V*, 1939, *47*, 23. See W. H. Sebrell and R. E. Butler, "Riboflavin Deficiency in Man," *Public Health Rep.*, 1938, *53*, 2282–84.

104. "Bishop Lawrence on Vivisection," *Living Tissue*, 1928, *13*, 5–6.

105. *The Menace of Human Vivisection* (Boston: New England Anti-Vivisection Society, 1926), p. 6.

106. Richard C. Cabot, "Medical Ethics in the Hospital," *Nosokomeion*, 1931, *2*, 158.

107. Ibid.

108. See "Use of Fifteen Year Old Boy as Skin Donor without Consent of Parents as Constituting Assault and Battery," *JAMA*, 1942, *120*, 562–63.

109. Bonner v. Moran, 75 U.S. App. D.C. 156, 126 F.2d 121 (1941).

Chapter Six

1. John C. Burnham, "American Medicine's Golden Age: What Happened to It?" *Science*, 1982, *215*, 1474–79.

2. Alphonse M. Schwitalla, "The Real Meaning of Research and Why It Should Be Encouraged," *Mod. Hosp.*, 1929, *32*, 79.

3. For an early battle with newspaper editors over the political meaning of self-experimentation, see "Fustian," *Animals' Defender*, 1902, *7*, 16–19.

4. Kenneth Ludmerer, *Learning to Heal: The Development of American Medical Education* (New York: Basic Books, 1985), pp. 208–11.

5. Stanley Joel Reiser, "Human Experimentation and the Convergence of Medical Research and Patient Care," *Annals AAPSS*, 1978, *437*, 8–18.

6. Rufus Cole, "Hospital and Laboratory," *Science*, 1927, *66*, 550.

7. Emmet B. Bay, "The Use of Paying Patients in Clinical Research and Teaching," *J. Assoc. Am. Med. Coll.*, 1946, *21*, 257–59.

8. "Refuse Permission to 'Revive' Dead Men," *New York Times*, 16 Oct. 1934; and Susan E. Lederer, "Laboratory Life on the Silver Screen: Animal Experimenters and the Film Industry in the 1930s and 40s," paper delivered at History of Science Society, Santa Fe, New Mexico, Nov. 1993.

9. The letters are discussed in Franc Dillon, "A Miracle Is Filmed," *Motion Picture*, Feb. 1935, pp. 40–41, 78–79.

10. Margarete J. Sandelowski, "Failures of Volition: Female Agency and Infertility in Historical Perspective," *Signs*, 1990, *15*, 495.

11. George Weisz, "The Posthumous Laennec: Creating a Modern Medical Hero, 1826–1870," *Bull. Hist. Med.*, 1987, *61*, 541–62.

12. "The Dangers of Pathologic Work," *JAMA*, 1907, *48*, 1112.

13. "Frozen While Making a Call," *JAMA*, 1929, *92*, 568.

14. P. Brown, *American Martyrs to Science through the Roentgen Rays* (Springfield, Ill.: Charles C. Thomas, 1936); F. G. Spears, "Radiation Martyrs," *Brit. J. Radiology*, 1956, *29*, 273.

15. "Obituary: Frederick Henry Baetjer," *JAMA*, 1933, *101*, 384.

16. Ruth and Edward Brecher, *The Rays: A History of Radiology in the United States and Canada* (Baltimore: Williams & Wilkins, 1969), pp. 171–73.

17. See "Another Martyr to Scientific Medicine—Thomas B. McClintic," *JAMA*, 1912, *59*, 550; Victoria A. Harden, *Rocky Mountain Spotted Fever: History of a Twentieth-Century Disease* (Baltimore: Johns Hopkins University Press, 1990), pp. 70–71; and Jerry K. Aikawa, *Rocky Mountain Spotted Fever* (Springfield, Ill.: Charles C. Thomas, 1966), p. 55.

18. See "Martyr to Study of Child Paralysis," *New York Times*, 5 Feb. 1933; and James N. Miller, "Test Tube Triumphs," *Hygeia*, 1941, 281–84.

19. "Research Woman Dies of Infection," *New York Times*, 27 Dec. 1935.

20. "Bacteriologist Dies of Meningitis," *JAMA*, 1936, *106*, 129.

21. Albert B. Sabin and A. M. Wright, "Acute Ascending Myelitis Following a Monkey Bite, With the Isolation of A Virus Capable of Reproducing the Disease," *J. Exp. Med.*, 1934, *59*, 115–36.

22. See "Psittacosis Has Attacked Eleven Laboratory Workers," *JAMA*, 1930, *94*, 1076; "Dr. Hasseltine Ill with Psittacosis for Second Time," *JAMA*, 1935, *105*, 727; "Dr. Meyer Ill with Psittacosis," *JAMA*, 1936, *106*, 47. Also see "Undulant Fever Contracted in Laboratory," *JAMA*, 1928, *91*, 1899.

23. Sterling Gleason, "Doctors Face Death Trailing Living Poisons of Mystery Diseases," *Popular Science Monthly*, 1933, *123*, 14.

24. Miller, "Test Tube Triumphs," p. 281.

25. Karl F. Meyer and B. Eddie, "Laboratory Infections Due to Brucella," *J. Infect. Dis.*, 1941, *68*, p. 29.

26. See Lucie Arvy, "Clara Louise Maass (1876–1901) et la Fièvre Jaune," *Clio Medica*, 1976, *13*, 277–82.

27. Wilbur A. Sawyer, "Recent Progress in Yellow Fever Research," *Medicine*, 1931, *10*, 531.

28. "Death of Prof. Adrian Stokes," *JAMA*, 1927, *89*, 1528.

29. "Dr. Noguchi is Dead, Martyr of Science," *New York Times*, 22 May 1928; "Martyrs of Medicine," *JAMA*, 1928, *90*, 1712–13; and "Another Martyr to Yellow Fever Research," *JAMA*, 1928, *91*, 107–8.

30. G. P. Berry and S. F. Kitchen, "Yellow Fever Accidentally Contracted in the Laboratory: A Study of Seven Cases," *Am. J. Trop. Med.*, 1931, *11*, 365.

31. Quote appears on cover of Paul de Kruif, *Microbe Hunters* (New York: Pocket Books, 1962). For de Kruif's role in the making of *Arrowsmith*, see Charles E. Rosenberg, "Martin Arrowsmith: The Scientist as Hero," in his *No Other Gods: On Science and American Social Thought* (Baltimore: Johns Hopkins University Press, 1976), pp. 123–32.

32. de Kruif, *Microbe Hunters*, p. 304.

33. Homer Croy, "Memories of a Yellow Fever Martyr," *The World's Work*, 1927, *55*, 151–57; and "Citizen's Committee Presents Home to Yellow Fever Volunteer," *JAMA*, 1927, *89*, 302.

34. Howard A. Kelly to W. W. Keen, 18 Dec. 1908, Keen Papers, CPP.

35. William W. Keen, *Animal Experimentation and Medical Progress* (Boston: Houghton Mifflin, 1914), p. 230.

36. Memorandum for Board of Directors, George Hoyt Whipple Papers, UR, box 3, f. 3.

37. "Grand Rapids Honors Yellow Fever Hero," *JAMA*, 1928, *91*, 733.

38. "Congress Honors the Yellow Fever Commission," *JAMA*, 1929, *92*, 984.

39. "Yellow Fever Volunteers Receive Congressional Medals," *JAMA*, 1931, *97*, 1718.

40. Quoted in "Again 'Yellow Jack,'" *Am. J. Pub. Health*, 1934, *24*, 651.

41. John J. Moran, *My Date with Walter Reed and "Yellow Jack,"* Hench Papers, UVA, box 60, f. 13. Also see Estelle Manette Raben, "*Men in White* and *Yellow Jack* as Mirrors of the Medical Profession," *Literature and Medicine*, 1993, *12*, 19–41.

42. "Yellow Jack," *The American Film Institute Catalog of Motion Pictures Produced in the United States, Feature Films, 1931–1940*, ed. Patricia King Hanson (Berkeley: University of California Press, 1993), p. 2481.

43. Ibid.

44. "Virginians Honor Yellow Fever Volunteer," *JAMA*, 1940, *115*, 1943; and "Memorial to Dr. Jesse Lazear," ibid., p. 1563.

45. "Medical History in Color," *Mil. Surg.*, 1941, *89*, 218–19.

46. Philip S. Hench, "Conquerors of Yellow Fever," *Hygeia*, 1941, *19*, 781–85.

47. Richard H. Shryock, *American Medical Research* (New York: Commonwealth Fund, 1947), p. 243.

48. Frank McVeigh to Louis B. Mayer, 13 Sept. 1938, Papers of the California Society for the Promotion of Medical Research, Ctn 1, UCSF.

49. See "Final Report of Campaign to Defeat the Proposed 'State Humane Pound Act' Initiative in California at the General Election—November 8, 1938," California Society for the Promotion of Medical Research Papers, UCSF. I am grateful to the Turner Entertainment Co. for providing me a viewing copy of the film.

50. "Correspondence," *The Starry Cross*, 1928, *37*, 140.

51. *How Vivisection Abolished Yellow Fever* in "Memorandum for Board of Directors," 25 Oct. 1927, George Hoyt Whipple Papers, UR, box 3, f. 3.

52. Virgil H. Moon, "What Price Antivivisection?" *Hygeia*, 1932, *10*, 1001.

53. "Heard and Read," *The Starry Cross*, 1935, *43*, 38. Also see "Exemplar," *The A-V*, 1942, *50*, 153.

54. A. W. Blair, "Spider Poisoning: Experimental Study of the Effects of the Bite of the Female Latrodectus Mactans in Man," *Arch. Int. Med.*, 1934, *54*, 831–43.

55. "Heard and Read," *The Starry Cross*, 1934, *42*, 115.

56. "Three Physicians Take New Serum in Test," *New York Times*, 6 July 1934.

57. Quoted in Harry Marks, "Notes from the Underground: The Social Organization of Therapeutic Research," in *Grand Rounds: One Hundred Years of Internal Medicine*, ed. Russell C. Maulitz and Diana E. Long (Philadelphia: University of Pennsylvania Press, 1988), p. 313.

58. "An Honest Doctor," *New Republic*, 1916, *9*, 246.

Epilogue

1. Albert T. Leffingwell, *An Ethical Problem*, 2nd ed., rev. (New York: C. P. Farrell, 1916), p. 325.

2. Henry K. Beecher, "Ethics and Clinical Research," *N. Eng. J. Med.*, 1966, *274*, 1354–60. See also Beecher's *Research and the Individual* (Boston: Little, Brown, 1970).

3. Michael A. Grodin and Joel J. Alpert, "Children as Participants in Medical Research," *Pediatr. Clin. North Am.*, 1988, *35*, 1389–1401.

4. David J. Rothman, *Strangers at the Bedside* (New York: Basic Books, 1991), pp. 30–50.

5. Ibid., p. 53.

6. George J. Annas and Michael A. Grodin, eds. *The Nazi Doctors and the Nuremberg Code* (New York: Oxford University Press, 1992).

7. James M. Jasper and Dorothy Nelkin, *The Animal Rights Crusade* (New York: Free Press, 1992), p. 70.

8. S. Wayman, "Concentration Camp for Dogs," *Life*, 4 Feb. 1966, pp. 22–29; see Andrew N. Rowan, *Of Mice, Molecules, and Men* (Albany: State University of New York Press, 1984), pp. 54–55.

9. Beecher, "Ethics and Clinical Research," p. 1356.

10. David J. Rothman, "Ethics and Human Experimentation: Henry Beecher Revisited," *N. Engl. J. Med.*, 1987, *317*, 1195–99.

11. Saul Krugman, "The Willowbrook Hepatitis Studies Revisited: Ethical Aspects," *Rev. Inf. Dis.*, 1986, *8*, 157–62; and Allan M. Brandt, "Racism and Research: The Case of the Tuskegee Syphilis Study," *Hastings Center Rep.*, 1978, *8*, 21–29.

12. Leffingwell, *An Ethical Problem*, p. 324.

Bibliographic Essay

Despite the interest in and controversy over using human subjects in medical research, historians have said comparatively little about human experimentation's role in the development of modern medicine, especially during the early part of the twentieth century, when clinical research became an integral part of scientific medicine. Some of the reasons for this gap in the historical literature are discussed in Gert H. Brieger's insightful essay, "Human Experimentation: History," in *Encyclopedia of Bioethics*, ed. Warren T. Reich (New York: Free Press, 1978), pp. 684–92. As Brieger maintains, going beyond a mere catalogue of human experiments requires knowledge not only of medical practice and medical science but of political, cultural, economic, and philosophical assumptions and conditions in society.

Several excellent case studies reflecting this comprehensive approach have been done in the last two decades. The most valuable relative to nineteenth-century medical science include: Edward C. Atwater, " 'Squeezing Mother Nature': Experimental Physiology in the United States before 1870," *Bull. Hist. Med.*, 1978, *52*, 313–35; Ronald L. Numbers, "William Beaumont and the Ethics of Human Experimentation," *J. Hist. Biol.*, 1979, *12*, 113–35; and Todd L. Savitt, "The Use of Blacks for Medical Experimentation and Demonstration in the Old South," *J. South. Hist.*, 1982, *48*, 331–48. Numbers's perceptive analysis of the moral dimensions of one of the best-known cases of human experimentation in American history—the man with the hole in his stomach, a case familiar to generations of American students—is a classic in the field. In a nuanced study of the relationship between white doctors and black subjects, Savitt emphasizes the vulnerability of black men and women at the hands of medical experimenters and medical educators. Also noteworthy as a case study of late-nineteenth and early-twentieth-century medical science is William B. Bean's "Walter Reed and the Ordeal of Human Experimentation," *Bull. Hist. Med.*, 1977, *51*, 75–92, which examines Reed's concerns about his subjects' welfare in the yellow fever research conducted in Cuba in 1900. Reed's ironic place in the history of human experimentation is also discussed in the ambitious survey by medical journalist Lawrence K. Altman, *Who Goes First? The Story of Self-Experimentation in Medicine* (New York: Random House, 1987).

For the growth and development of clinical trials, a significant feature of twentieth-century human experimentation, a valuable starting place is the essay by Harry M. Marks, "Notes from the Underground: The Social Organization of Therapeutic Research," in *Grand Rounds: One Hundred Years of Internal Medicine,* ed. Russell C. Maulitz and Diana E. Long (Philadelphia: University of Pennsylvania Press, 1988), pp. 297–336. Marks emphasizes how clinical researchers in the 1930s and 1940s conceived of controlled clinical studies before they had the social and organizational strategies to conduct them successfully.

Indispensable for understanding the longest nontherapeutic human experiment in the history of twentieth-century medical science are Allan M. Brandt, "Racism and Research: The Case of the Tuskegee Syphilis Study," *Hastings Center Rep.*, 1978, *8*, 21–29, and the monograph by James H. Jones, *Bad Blood: The Tuskegee Syphilis Experiment* (New York: Free Press, 1981). The history of how the Tuskegee Syphilis Study and a number of other scandalous human experiments produced, in the 1970s, the first federal regulations for the protection of human subjects is perceptively analyzed in David J. Rothman's *Strangers at the Bedside: A History of How Law and Bioethics Transformed Medical Decision Making* (New York: Basic Books, 1991).

The history of human experimentation cannot be understood independently of the development of ideas about informed consent for medical treatment. Two important sources for this aspect of medical practice are: Martin Pernick's essay, "The Patient's Role in Medical Decisionmaking: A Social History of Informed Consent in Medical Therapy," in President's Commission for the Study of Ethical Problems in Medicine and Biomedical and Behavioral Research, *Making Health Care Decisions* (Washington, D.C.: Government Printing Office, 1982), vol. 3; and Ruth R. Faden and Tom L. Beauchamp, *A History and Theory of Informed Consent* (New York: Oxford University Press, 1986).

Bioethicists have made important contributions to the understanding of the recent history of human experimentation. A rich source of information for the international context of human subjects research in the twentieth century is *The Nazi Doctors and the Nuremberg Code: Human Rights in Human Experimentation*, ed. George J. Annas and Michael A. Grodin (New York: Oxford University Press, 1992). Annas's essay, "The Nuremberg Code in U.S. Courts: Ethics versus Expediency," is especially significant for focusing scholarly attention on the legal history of human experimentation in the American context. Historical dimensions of the special problems posed by experimentation involving children are explored in Susan E. Lederer and Michael A. Grodin's "Historical Overview," in *Children as Research Subjects: Science, Ethics, and Law* (New York: Oxford University Press, 1994), pp. 3–28, and in Susan E. Lederer, "Orphans as Guinea Pigs: American Children and Medical Experimenters, 1890–1930," in *In the Name of the Child: Health and Welfare, 1880–1940*, ed. Roger Cooter (London: Routledge, 1992), pp. 96–123.

Just as public interest in human experimentation fostered greater scholarly interest in the history of human experimentation, the rise of the animal rights movement has produced a growing literature on the history of animal protection and antivivisection. Although some work has been done, the history of animal experimentation in America, as such, remains to be written. The opposition to animal experimentation has initially attracted greater interest from historians. Essential reading on the British movement against animal experimentation is Richard D. French, *Antivivisection and Medical Science in Victorian Society* (Princeton: Princeton University Press, 1975). For a comparison between the British and American animal protection movements, see James C. Turner, *Reckoning with the Beast: Animals, Pain, and Humanity in the Victorian Mind* (Baltimore: Johns Hopkins University Press, 1980). A recent collection of essays, *Vivisection in Historical Perspective*, ed. Nicolaas A. Rupke (London: Croom Helm, 1987), offers new perspectives on the history of both British and American antivivisectionism. Two essays in the Rupke volume are especially useful: Christopher Lawrence, " 'Cinema Vérité?' The Image of William Harvey's Experiments in 1928," and Mary Ann Elston's "Women and Anti-Vivisection in Victorian England, 1870–1900." Lawrence's essay is one of the few to bring the antivivisection movement into the twentieth century, especially into the critical period between the two world wars.

The links between the antivivisectionist and other reform movements in the nineteenth century still need to be worked out. For the child welfare movement, Linda Gordon's *Heroes of Their Own Lives: The Politics and History of Family Violence, Boston 1880–1960* (New York: Viking Press, 1988) is a good starting place. For the temperance movement, see Ruth Bordin, *Wom-*

an and Temperance: The Quest for Power and Liberty, 1873–1900 (Philadelphia: Temple University Press, 1981), and Philip J. Pauly, "The Struggle for Ignorance about Alcohol: American Physiologists, Wilbur Olin Atwater, and the Woman's Christian Temperance Union," *Bull. Hist. Med.*, 1990, *64*, 366–92.

The other important context for understanding the American antivivisection movement is the development of medical research in the United States. Richard H. Shryock's *American Medical Research Past and Present* (New York: Commonwealth Fund, 1947) remains an effective starting point. On the nineteenth-century origins of scientific medicine, John Harley Warner, *The Therapeutic Perspective: Medical Practice, Knowledge, and Identity in America, 1820–1885* (Cambridge: Harvard University Press, 1986) must not be overlooked. Important sources for the twentieth century include: George W. Corner's *A History of the Rockefeller Institute* (New York: Rockefeller Institute Press, 1964); Victoria A. Harden, *Inventing the NIH: Federal Biomedical Research Policy, 1887–1937* (Baltimore: Johns Hopkins University Press, 1986); and A. McGehee Harvey, *Science at the Bedside: Clinical Research in American Medicine, 1905–1945* (Baltimore: Johns Hopkins University Press, 1981).

Biographies of significant researchers are another useful aid in understanding the reciprocal influence of antivivisection on medical science in the late nineteenth century and the twentieth century. One biography essential to understanding the antivivisection movement is Saul Benison, A. Clifford Barger, and Elin L. Wolfe, *Walter B. Cannon: The Life and Times of a Young Scientist* (Cambridge: Harvard University Press, 1987), which traces Cannon's pivotal role in the American battles over laboratory animal protection. I have discussed Cannon's role in the history of human and animal experimentation in "'The Right and Wrong of Making Experiments on Human Beings': Udo J. Wile and Syphilis, 1916," *Bull. Hist. Med.*, 1984, *58*, 380–97; and "Hideyo Noguchi's Luetin Experiment and the Antivivisectionists," *Isis*, 1985, *76*, 31–48.

Index

Library of Congress Cataloging-in-Publication Data

Lederer, Susan E.
  Subjected to science: human experimentation in America
before the Second World War / Susan E. Lederer.
      p.   cm. — (Henry E. Sigerist series in the history of
medicine)
  Includes bibliographical references and index.
  ISBN 0-8018-4820-2 (hc : alk. paper)
  1. Human experimentation in medicine—United States—
History—20th century. I. Title. II. Series.
  [DNLM: 1. Human Experimentation—history—United
States.   WZ 70 AA1 L4s 1995]
R853.H8L43   1994
174'.28—dc20
DNLM/DLC
for Library of Congress   94-27816